Princess of Chair

Vol.1

Farnaz Bordbar

Vancouver, BC CANADA

Copyright © 2024 by Kashti Nooh Publishing Inst.

All rights reserved. No part of this publication may be reproduced, distributed or transmitted in any form or by any means, including photocopying, recording, or other electronic or mechanical methods, without the prior written permission of the publisher, except in the case of brief quotations embodied in critical reviews and certain other noncommercial uses permitted by copyright law. For permission requests, write to the publisher, addressed "Attention: Permissions Coordinator," at the address below.

Published by: Kashti Nooh Publishing Inst.

Vancouver, BC **CANADA**
Email: Info@kashtinooh.com
www.kashtinooh.com

Ordering Information:
Quantity sales. Special discounts are available on quantity purchases by universities, schools, corporations, associations, and others. For details, contact the "Sales Department" at the above mentioned email address.

Princess of Chair, Vol.1 /Farnaz Bordbar—1st. ed.
ISBN: 978-1-77899-007-6   Paperback

Every possible effort has been made to ensure that the information contained in this book is accurate at the time of going to press, and the publishers and the author cannot accept responsibility for any errors or omissions, however caused. No responsibility for loss or damage occasioned to any person acting, or refraining from action, as a result of the material in this publication can be accepted by the publisher and/or the author.

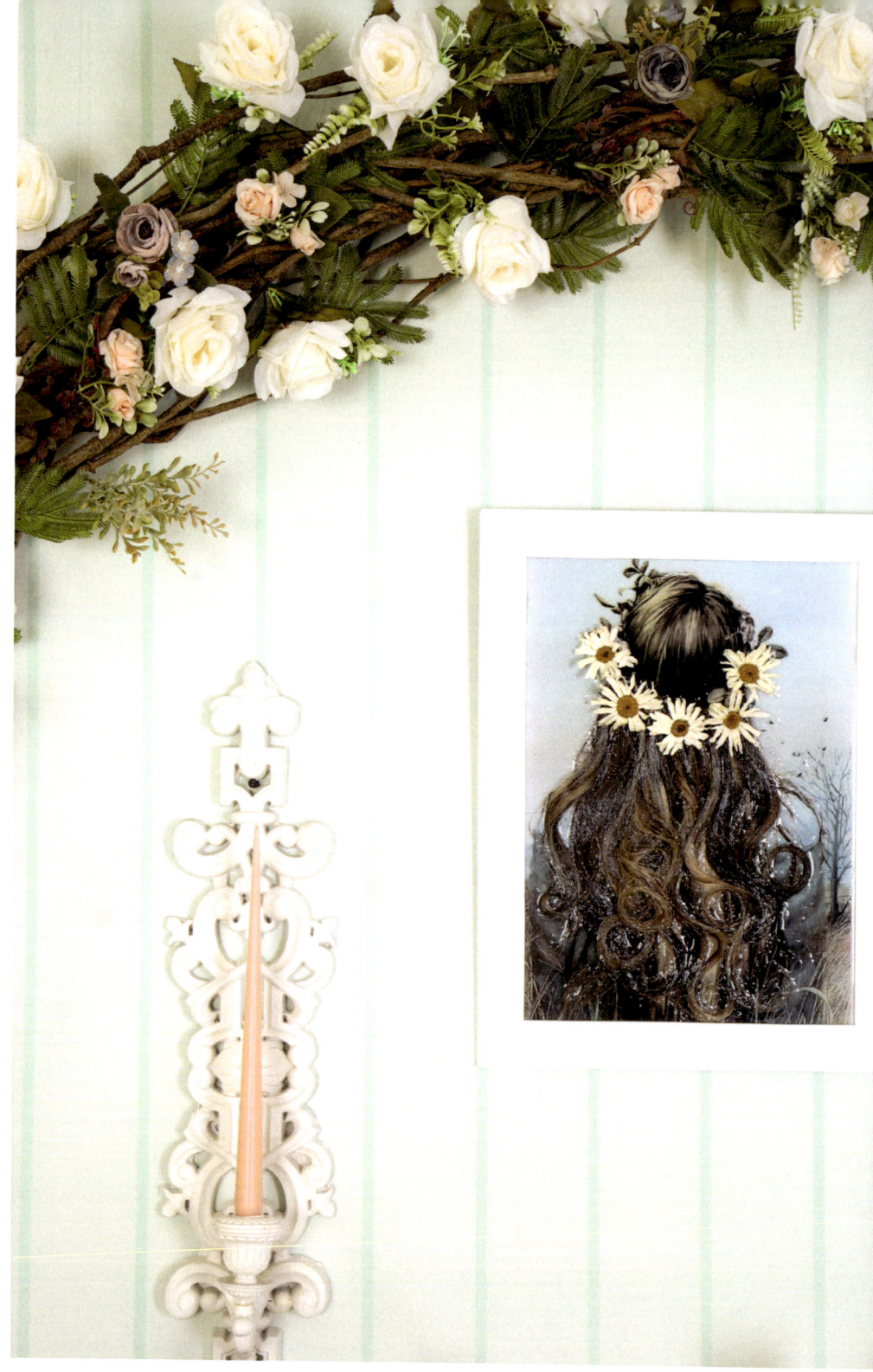

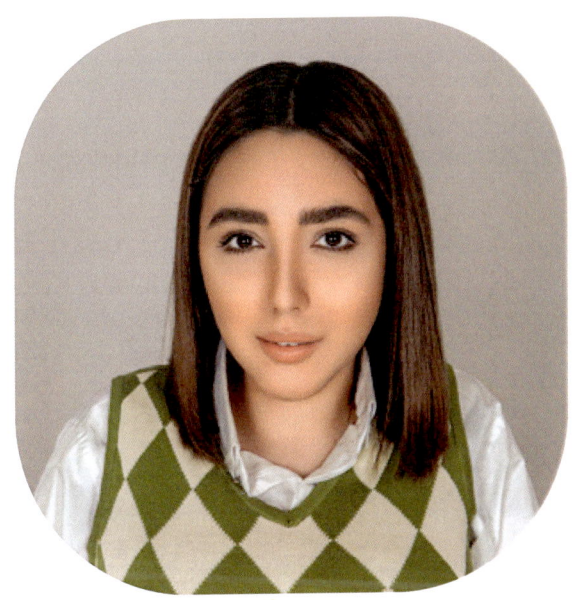

Farnaz Bordbar

is a model with a unique sense of style...
She has a bachelor's degree in English translation... She was born on December 1, 1991 in Iran, where there are numerous limitations in regard to female modeling...
Farnaz was diagnosed with a rare genetic condition called SMA, which left her paralyzed at the age 2. Despite the tremendous challenges she faces, not only has she survived but she has also thrived to pursue her passion...
At the age of 25, with the invention of spinraza medication, she aspired to find her place in an international scale and be influential for upcoming generations...
She mastered a distinctive style in creating her art and loves her family, which she believes has constantly inspired her to become better and more professional. Farnaz is also motivated to create a brighter and happier life for the future generations...

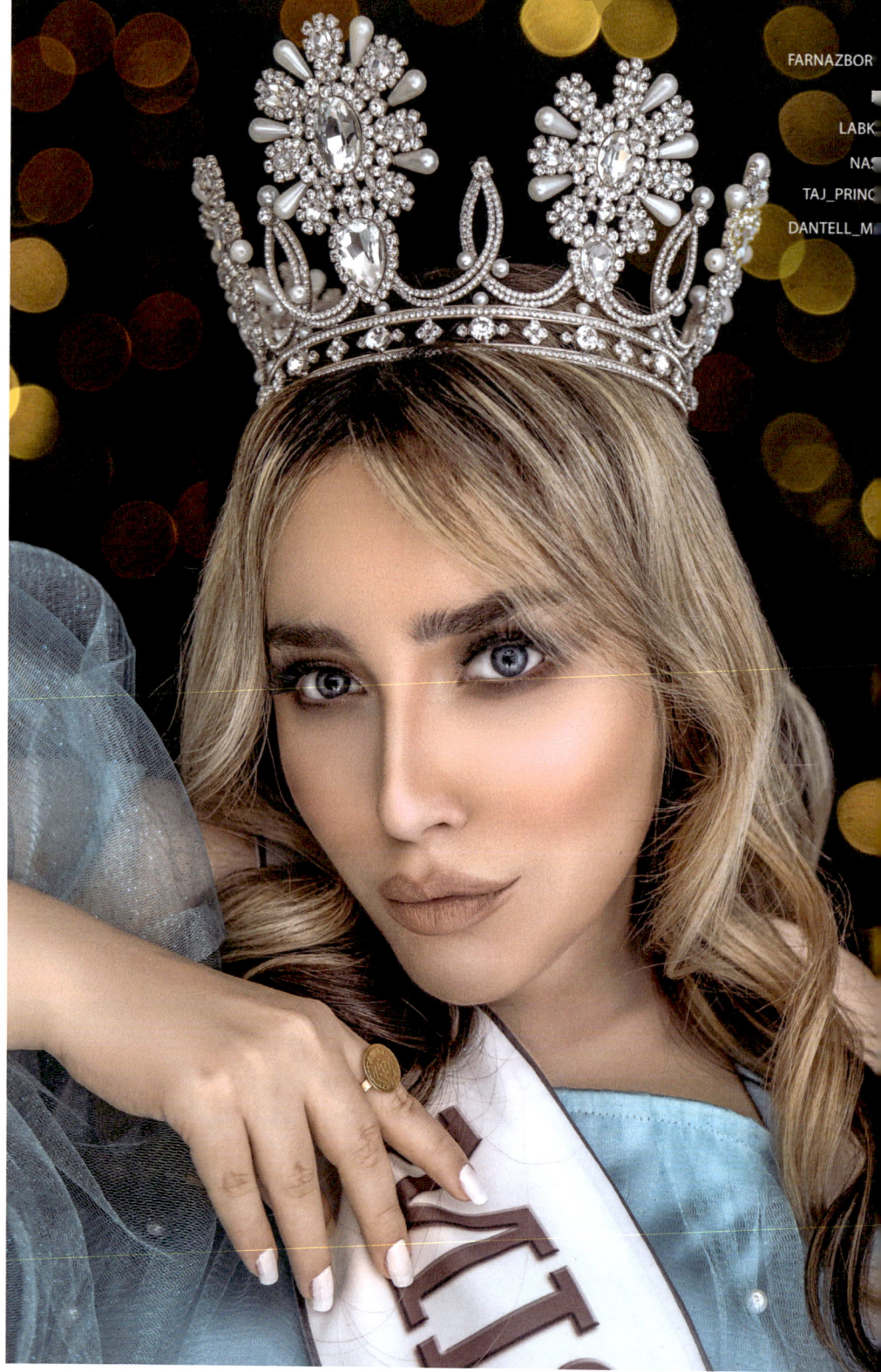

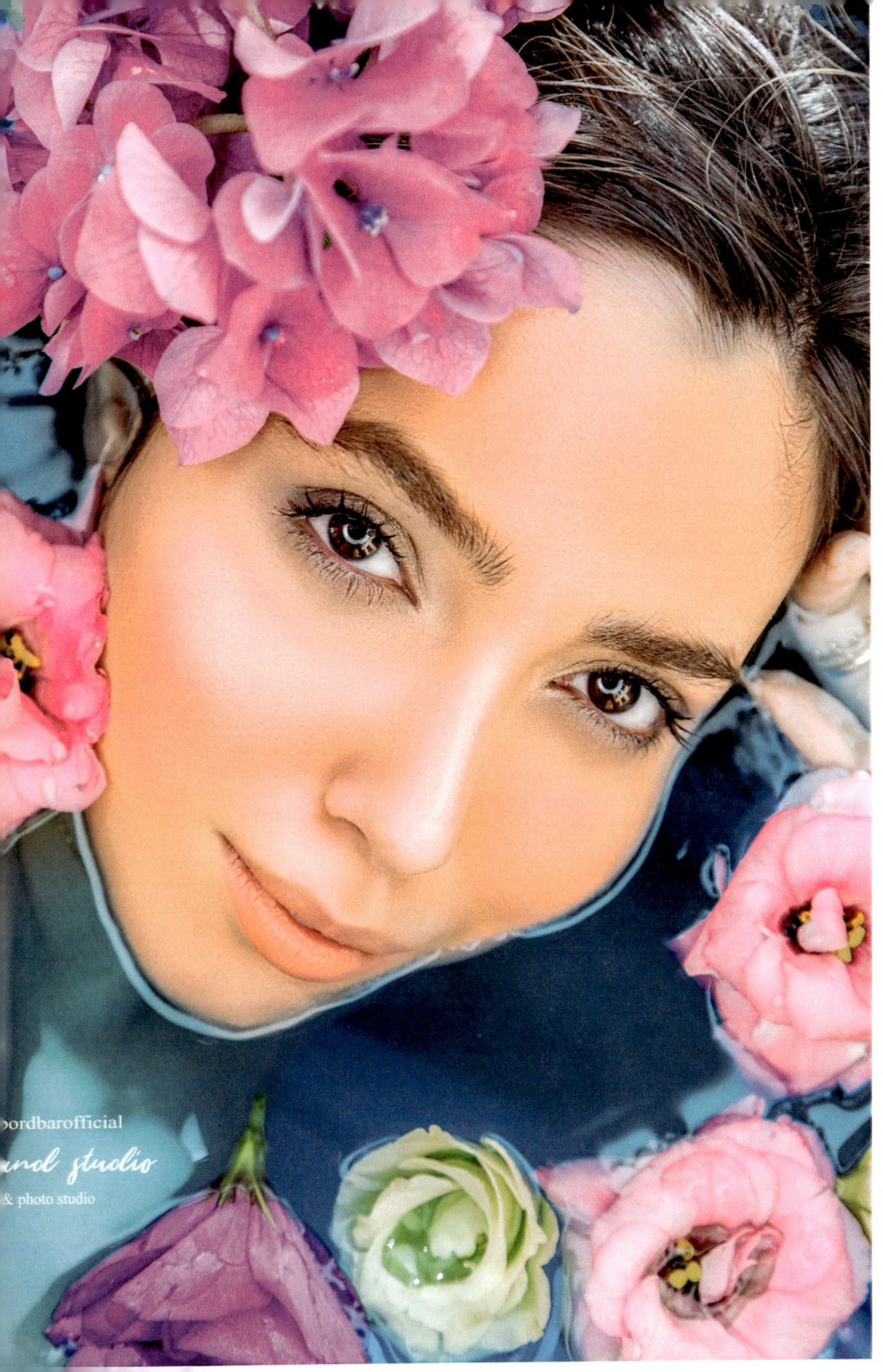

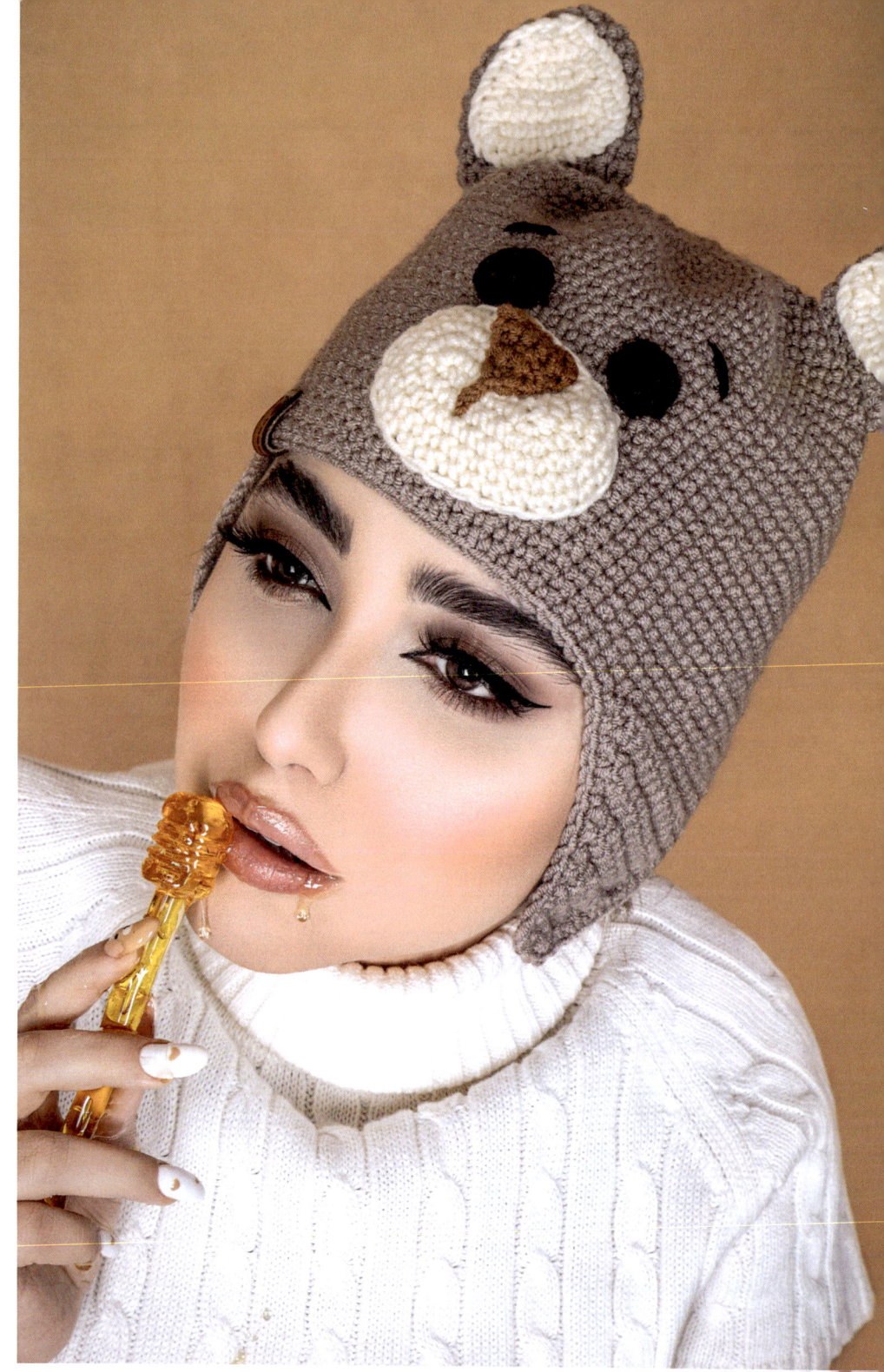

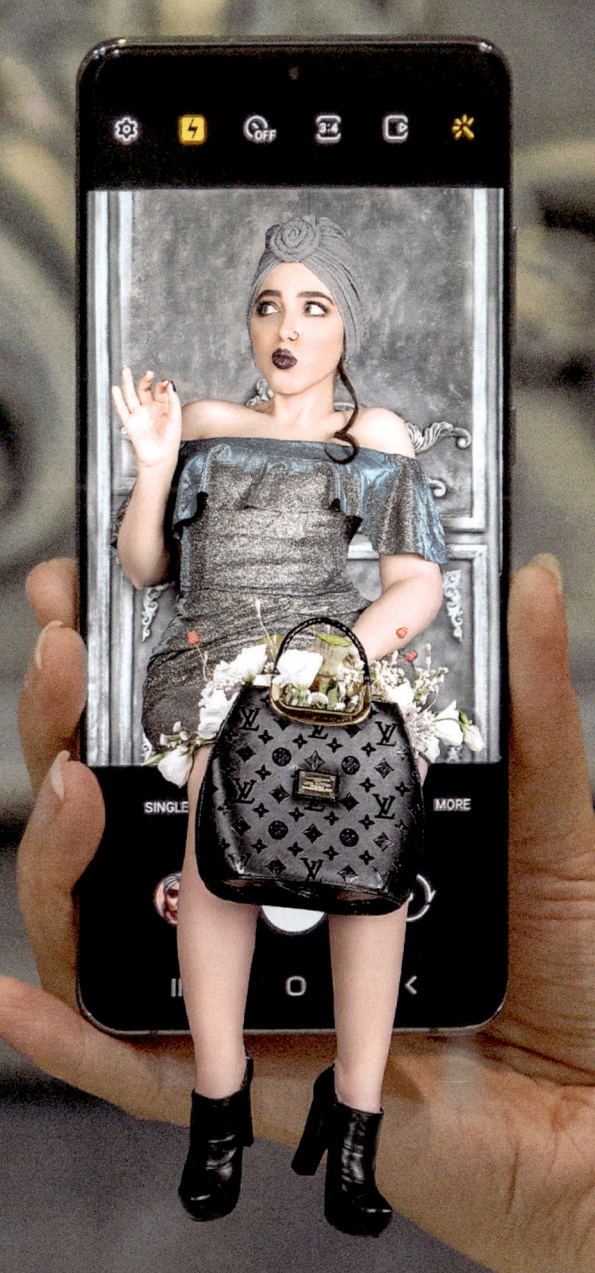

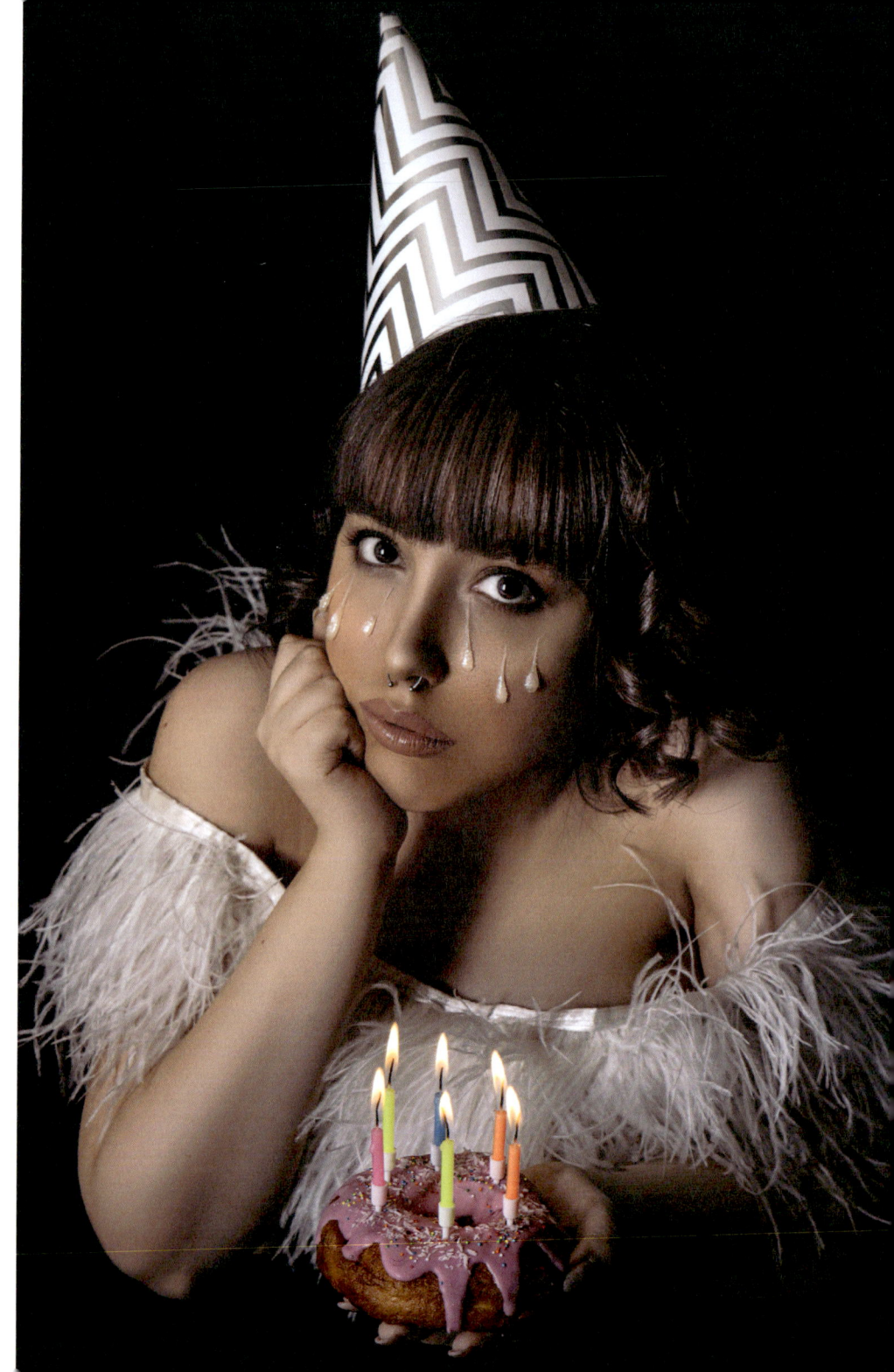

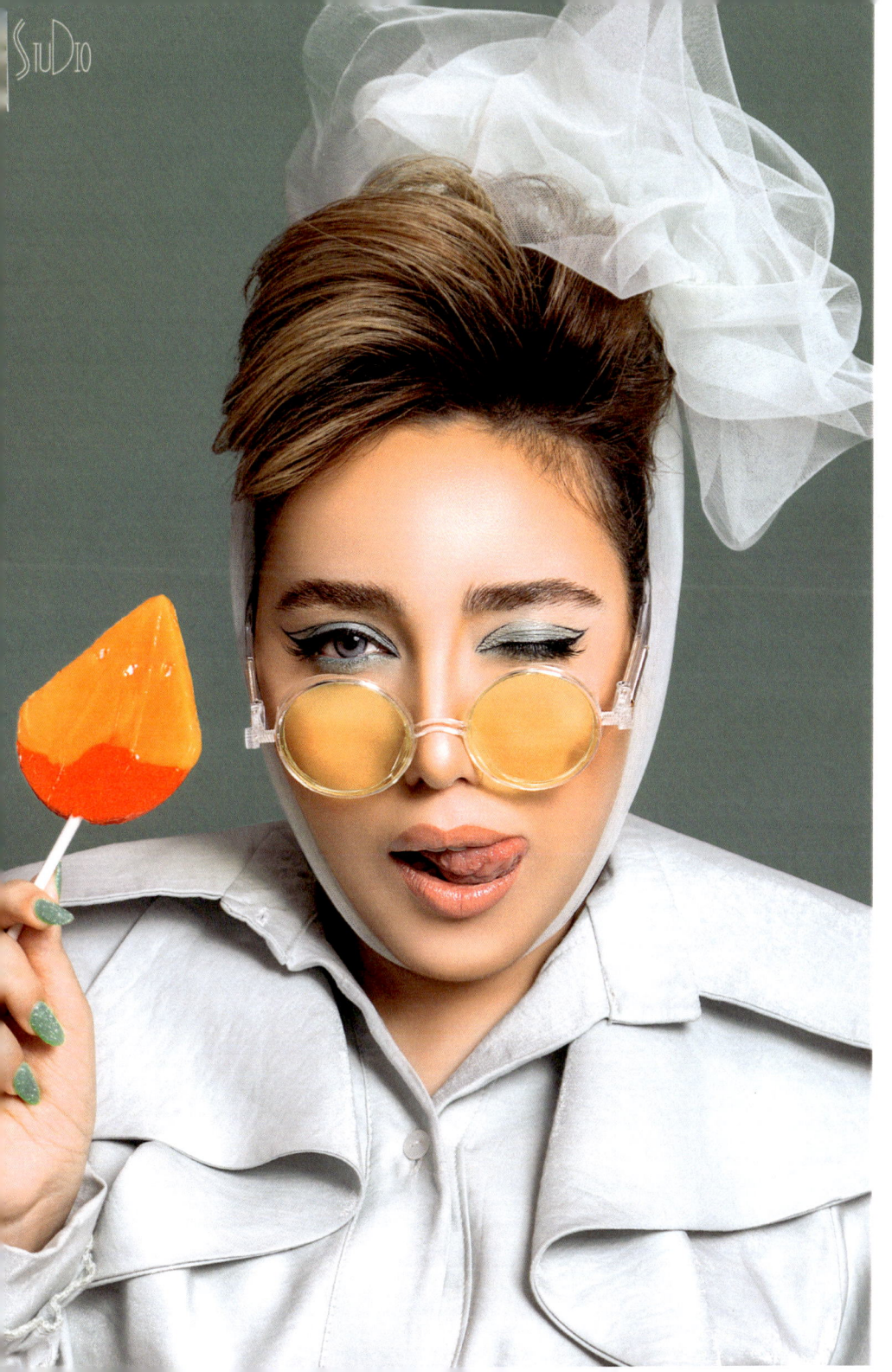

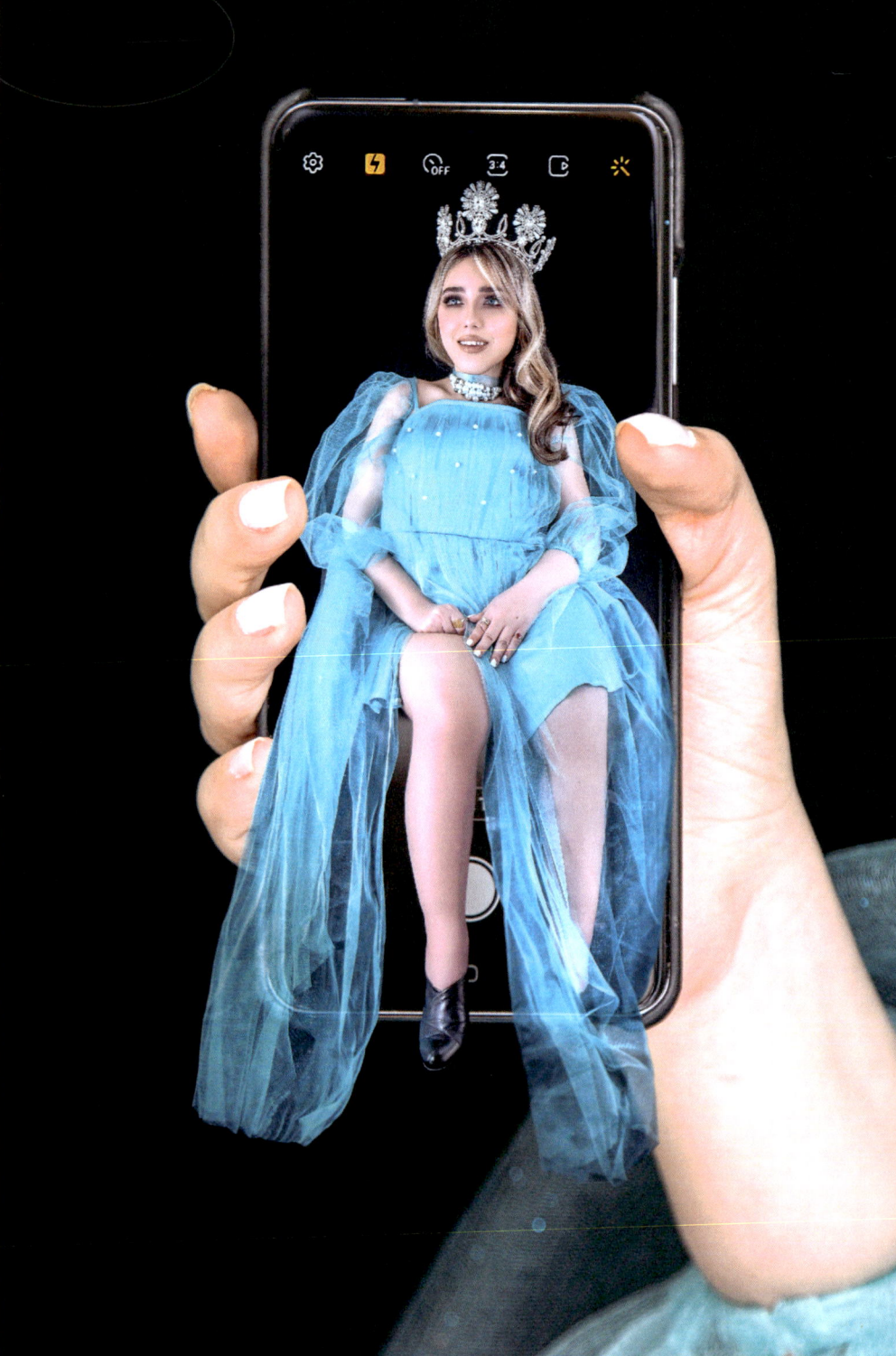

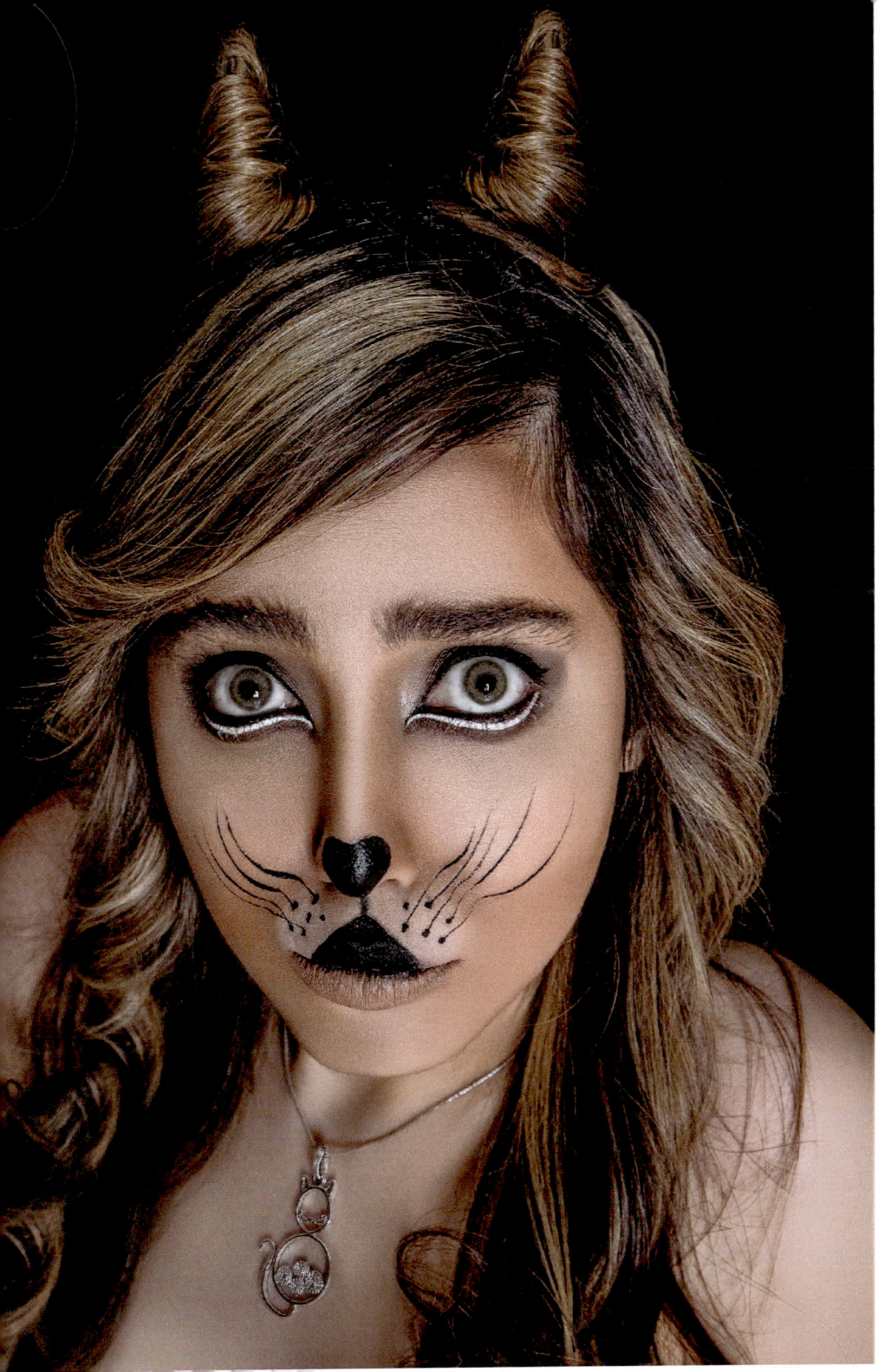

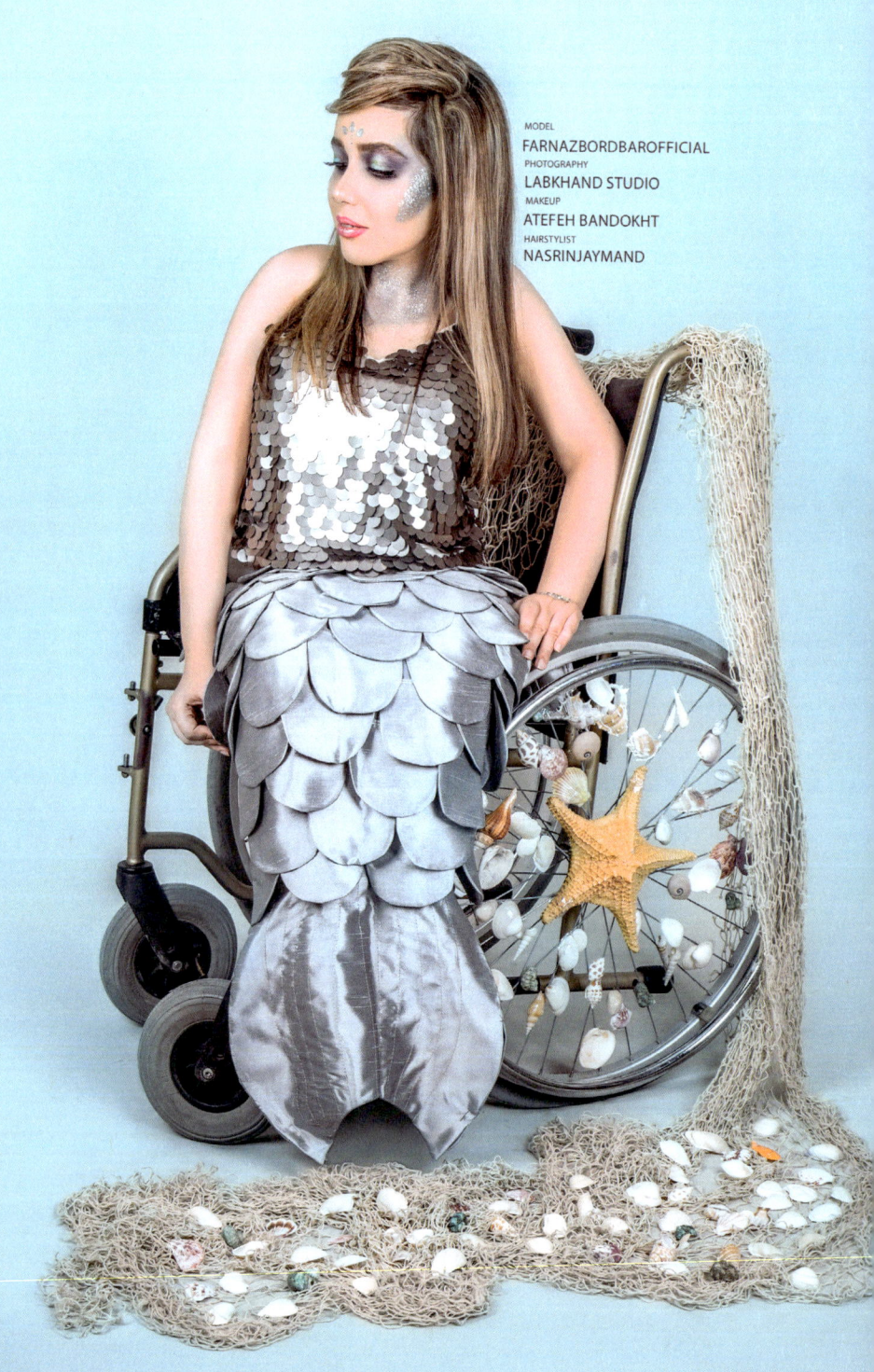

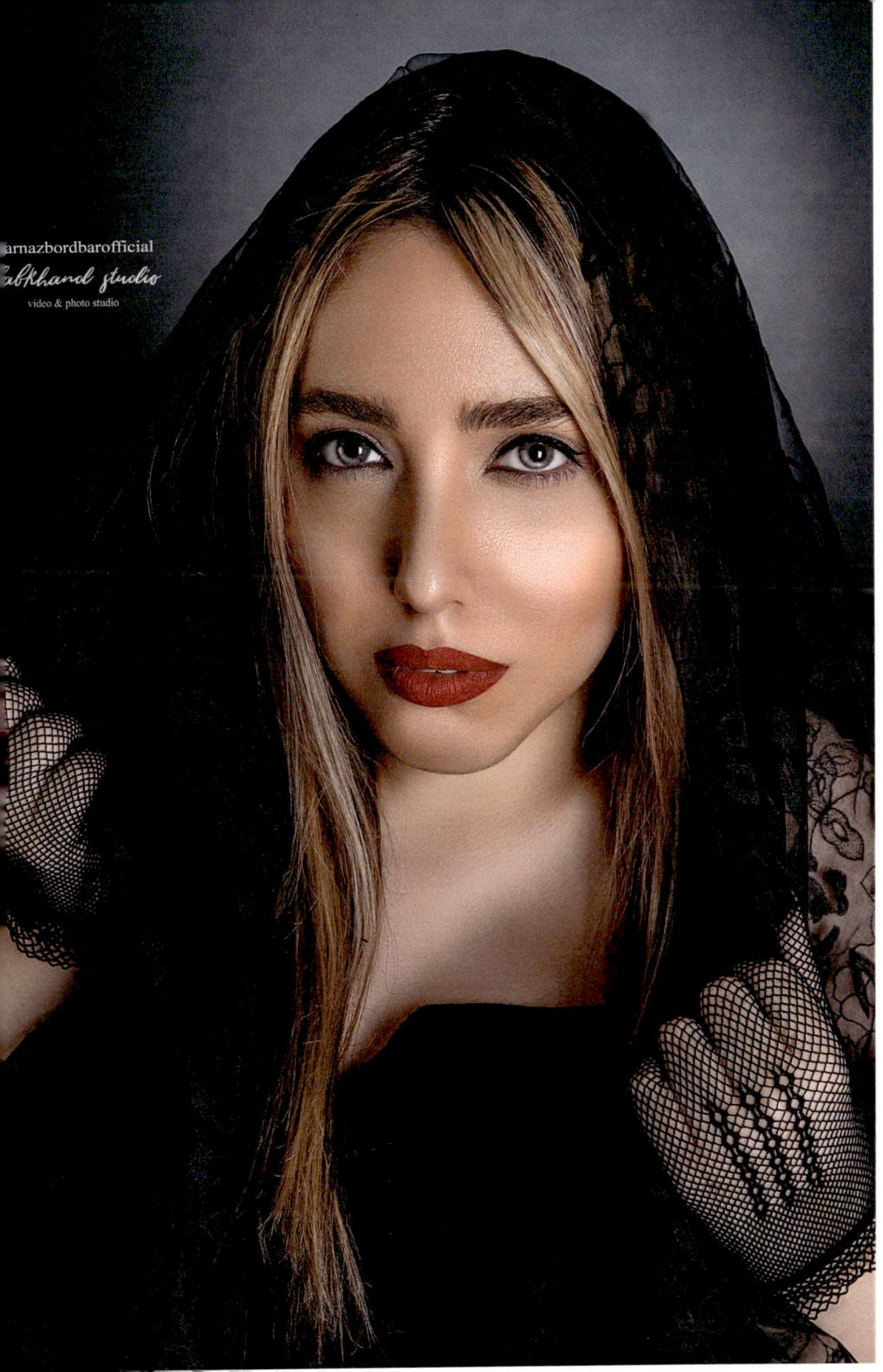

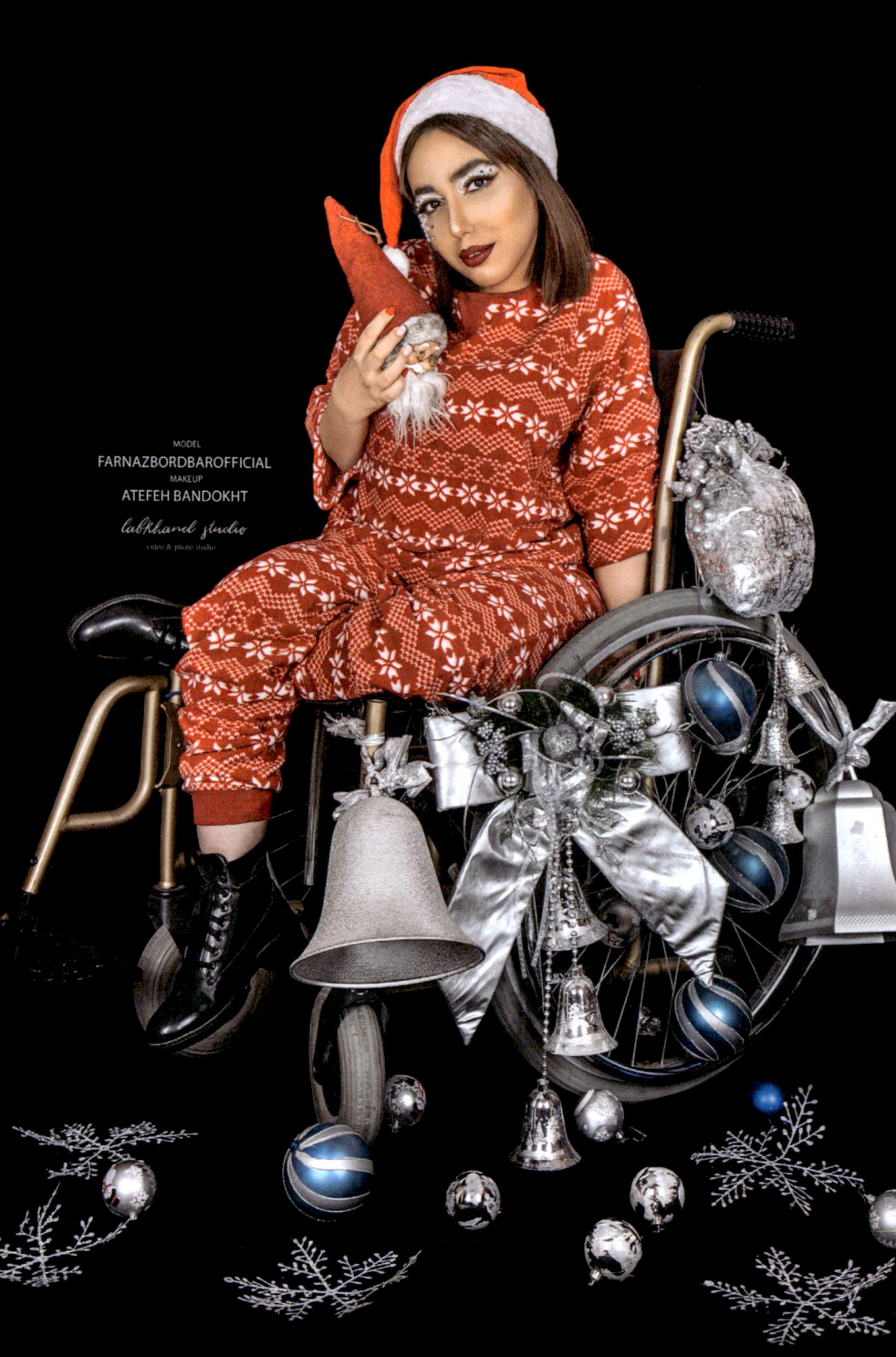

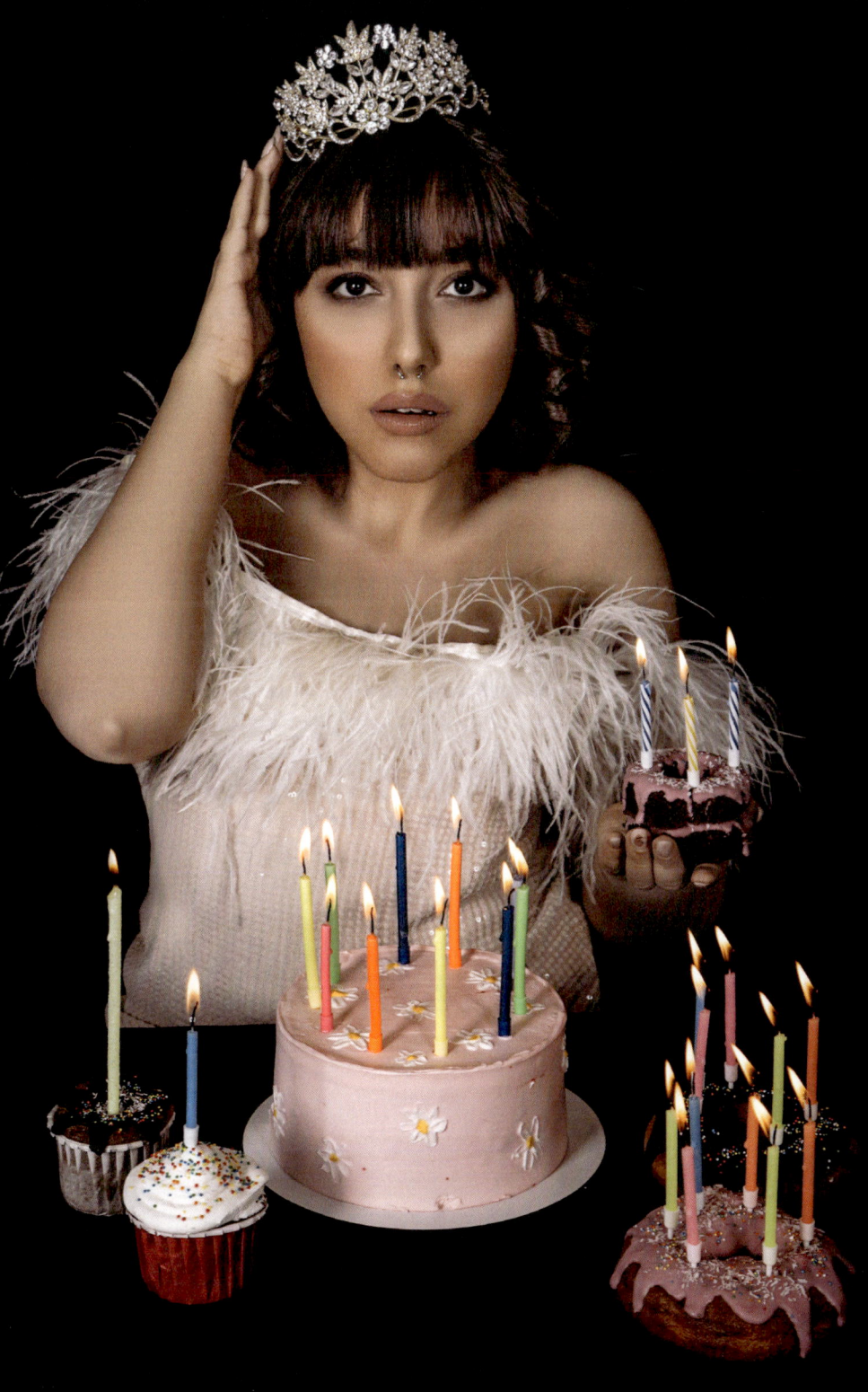

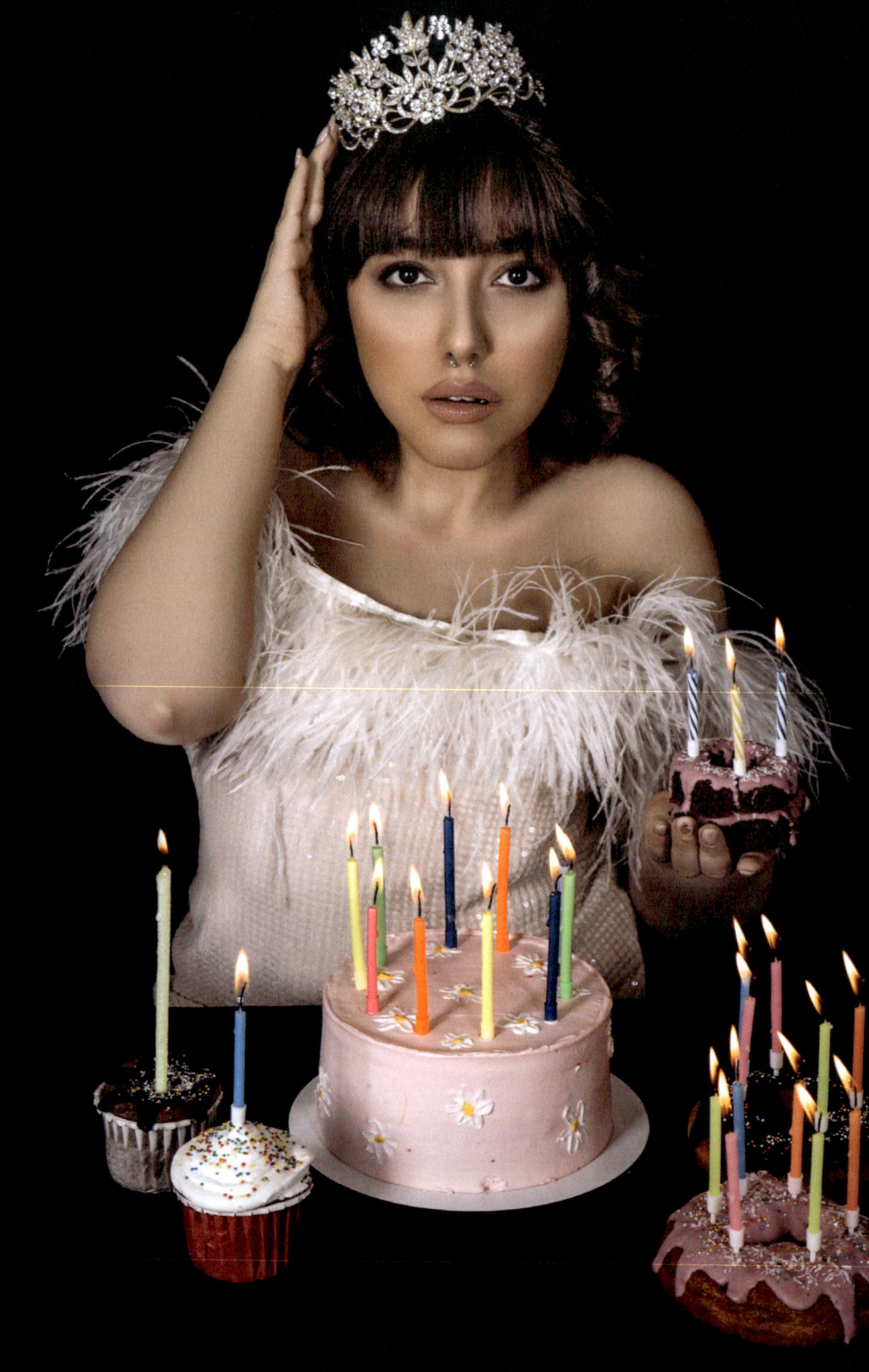

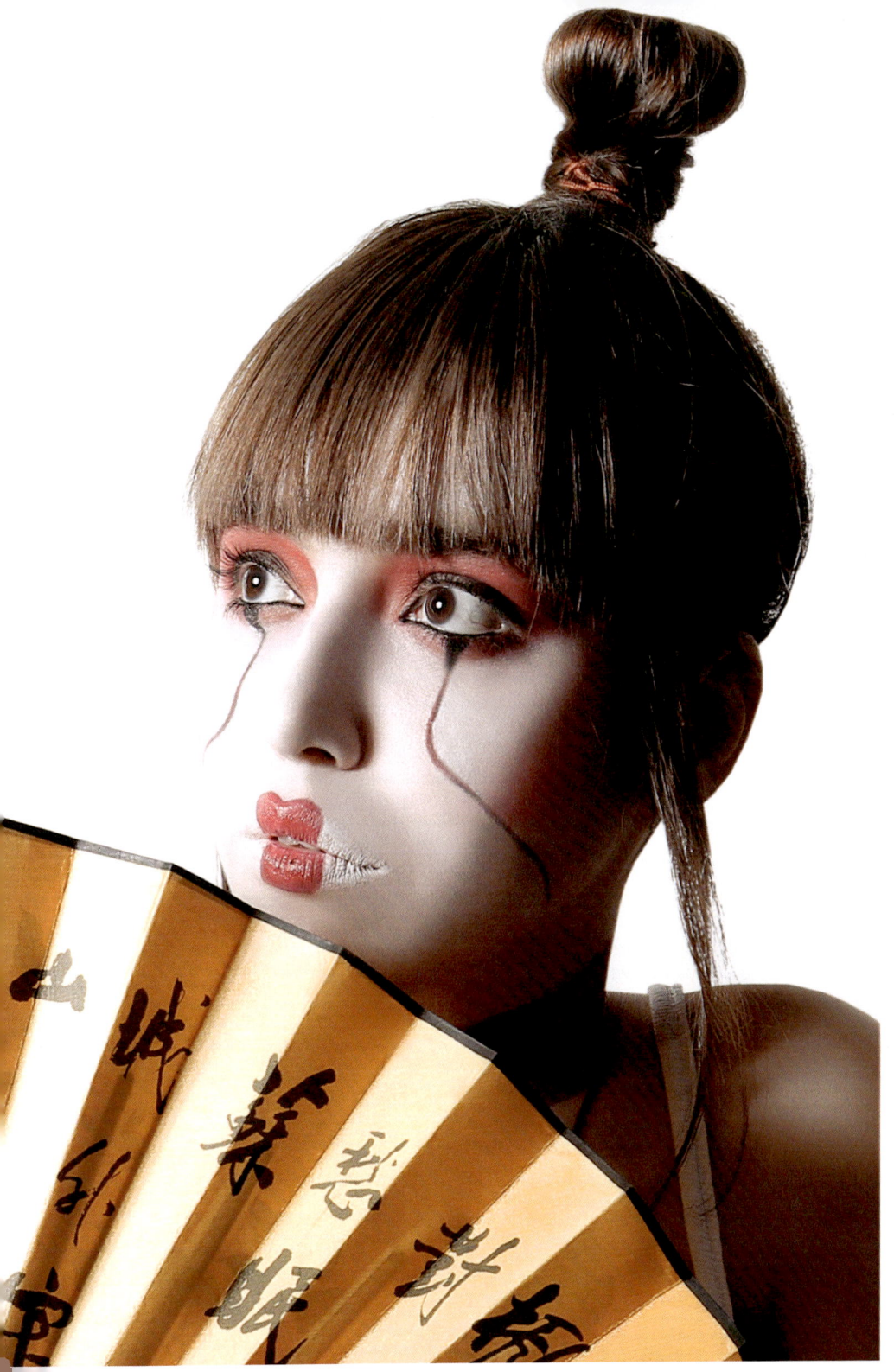

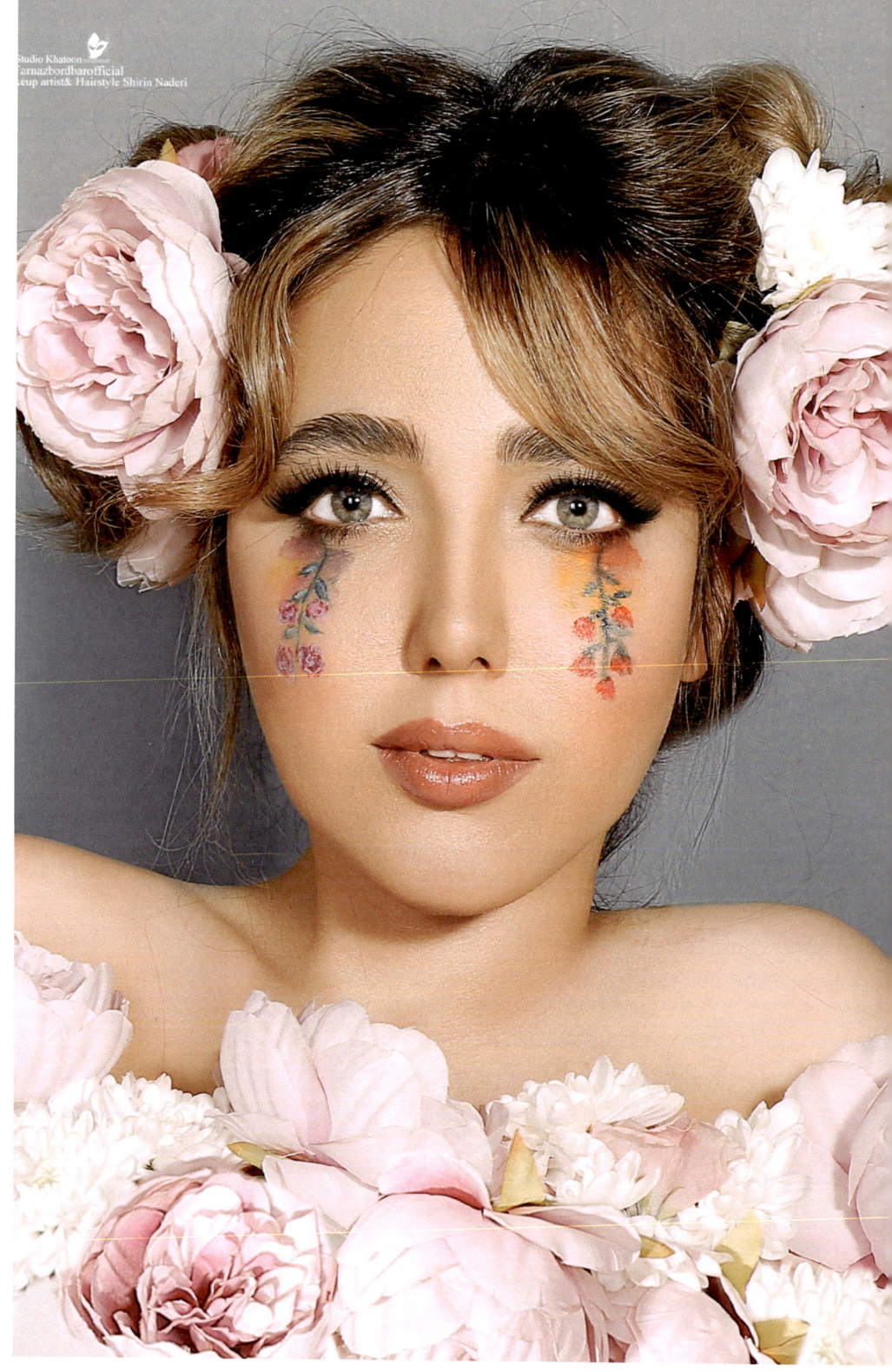

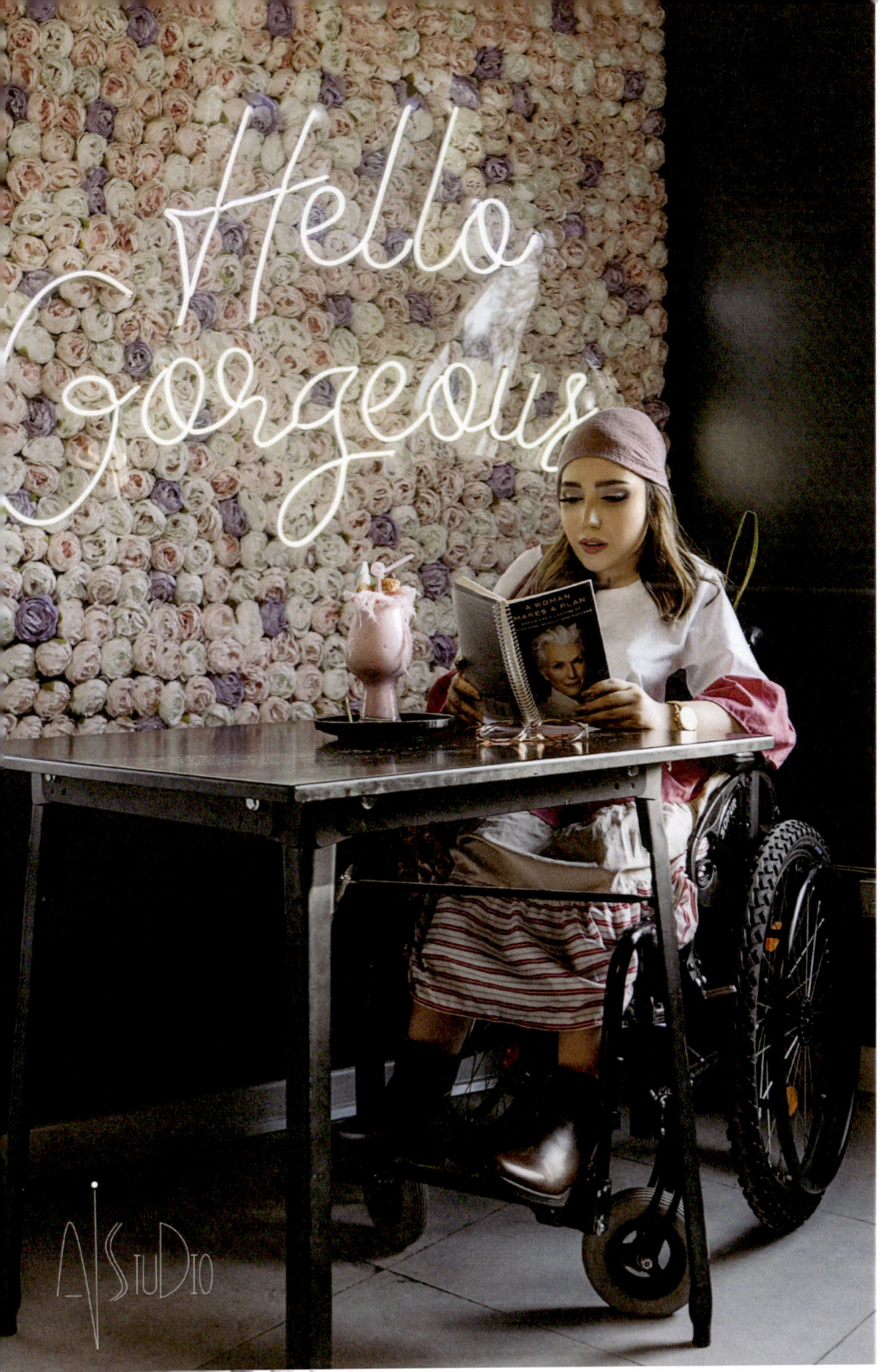

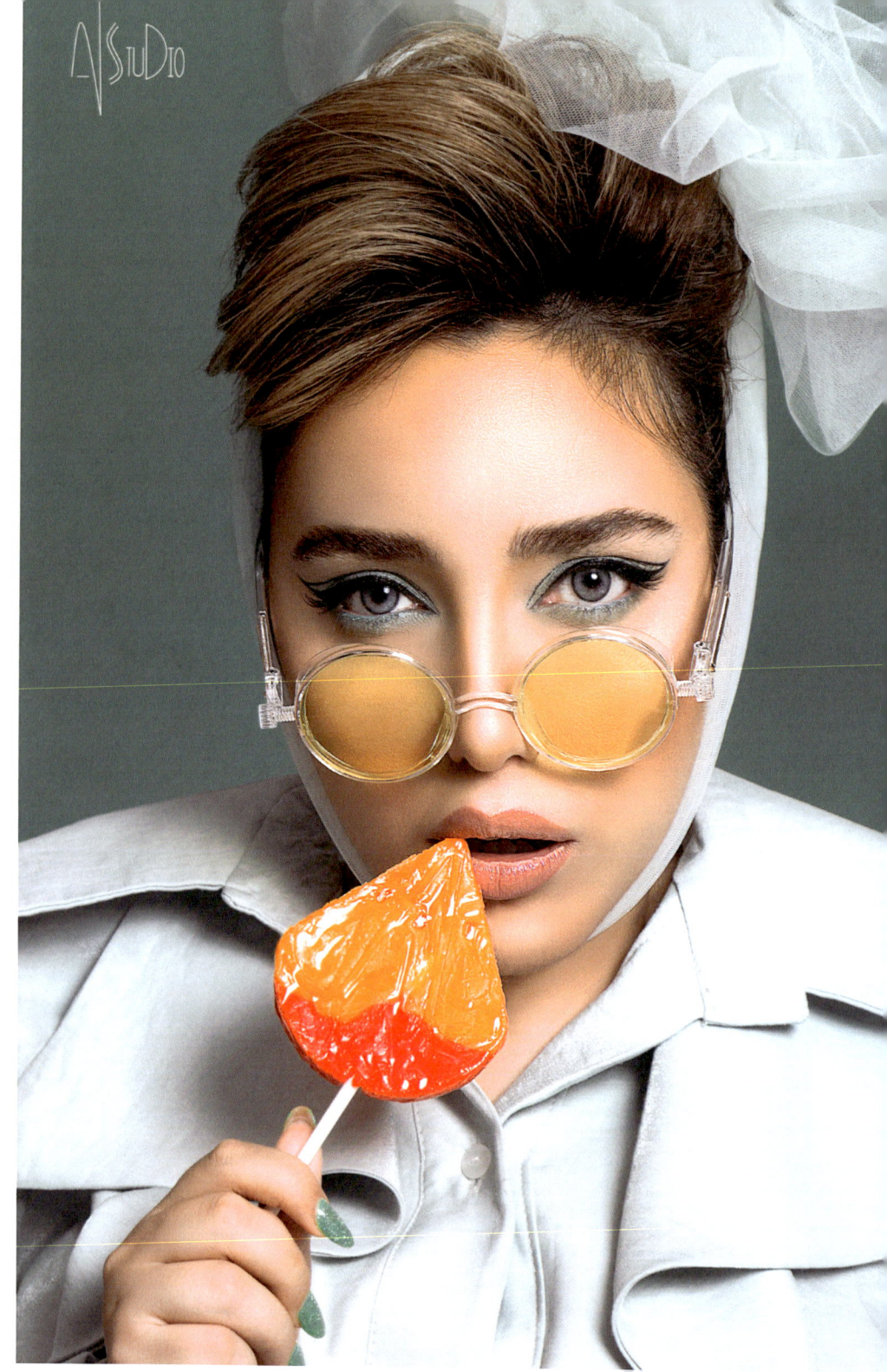

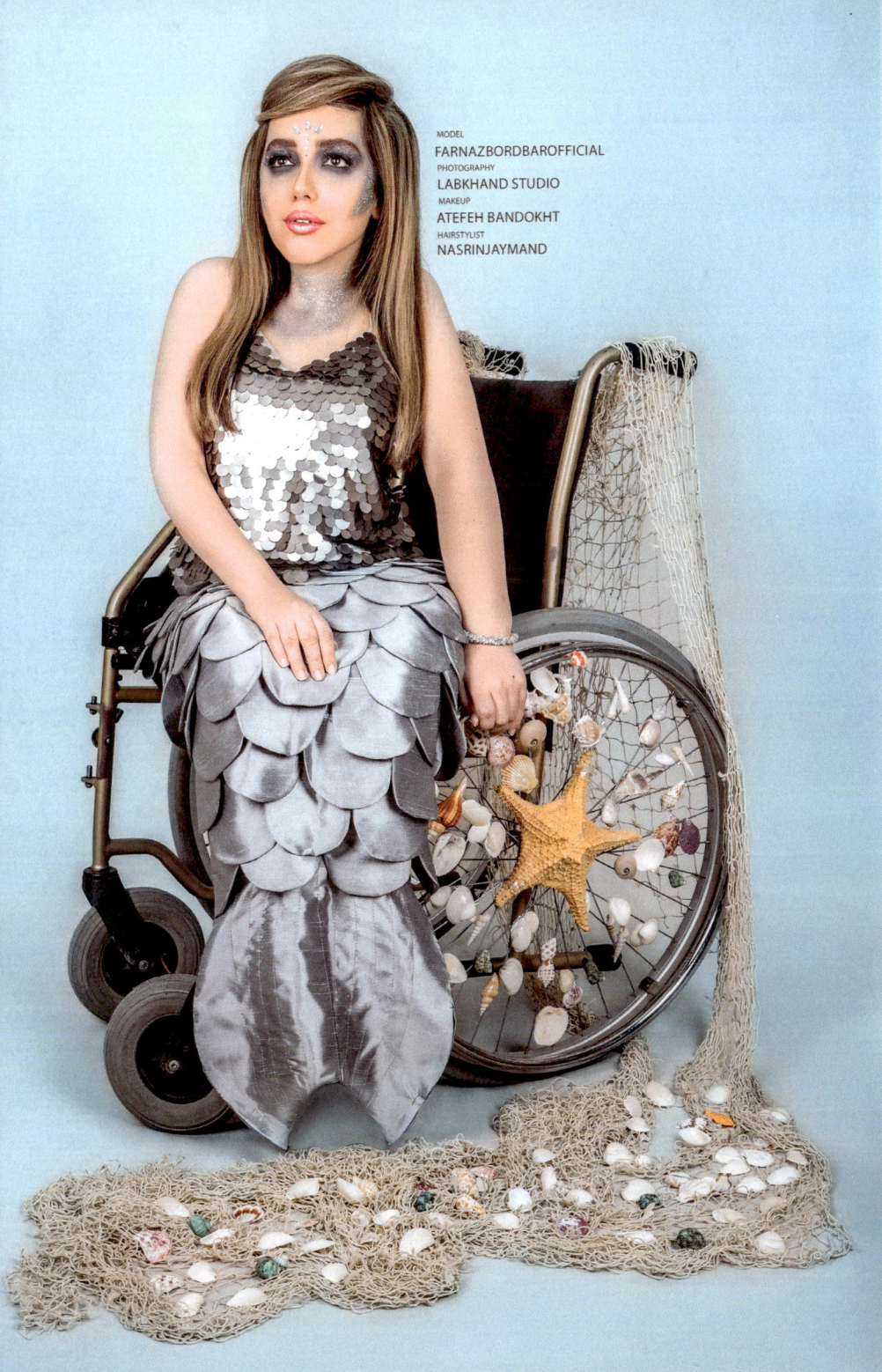

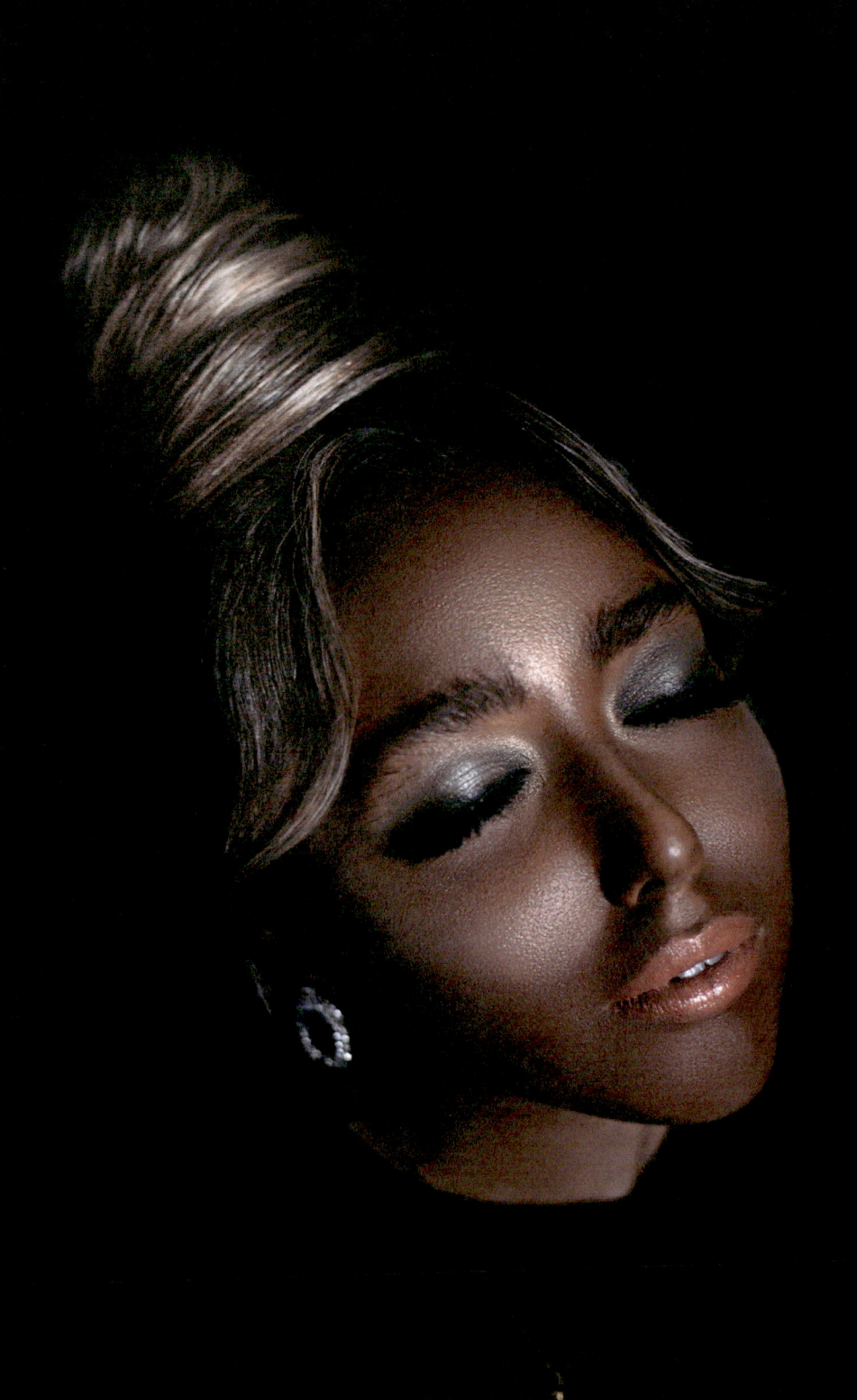

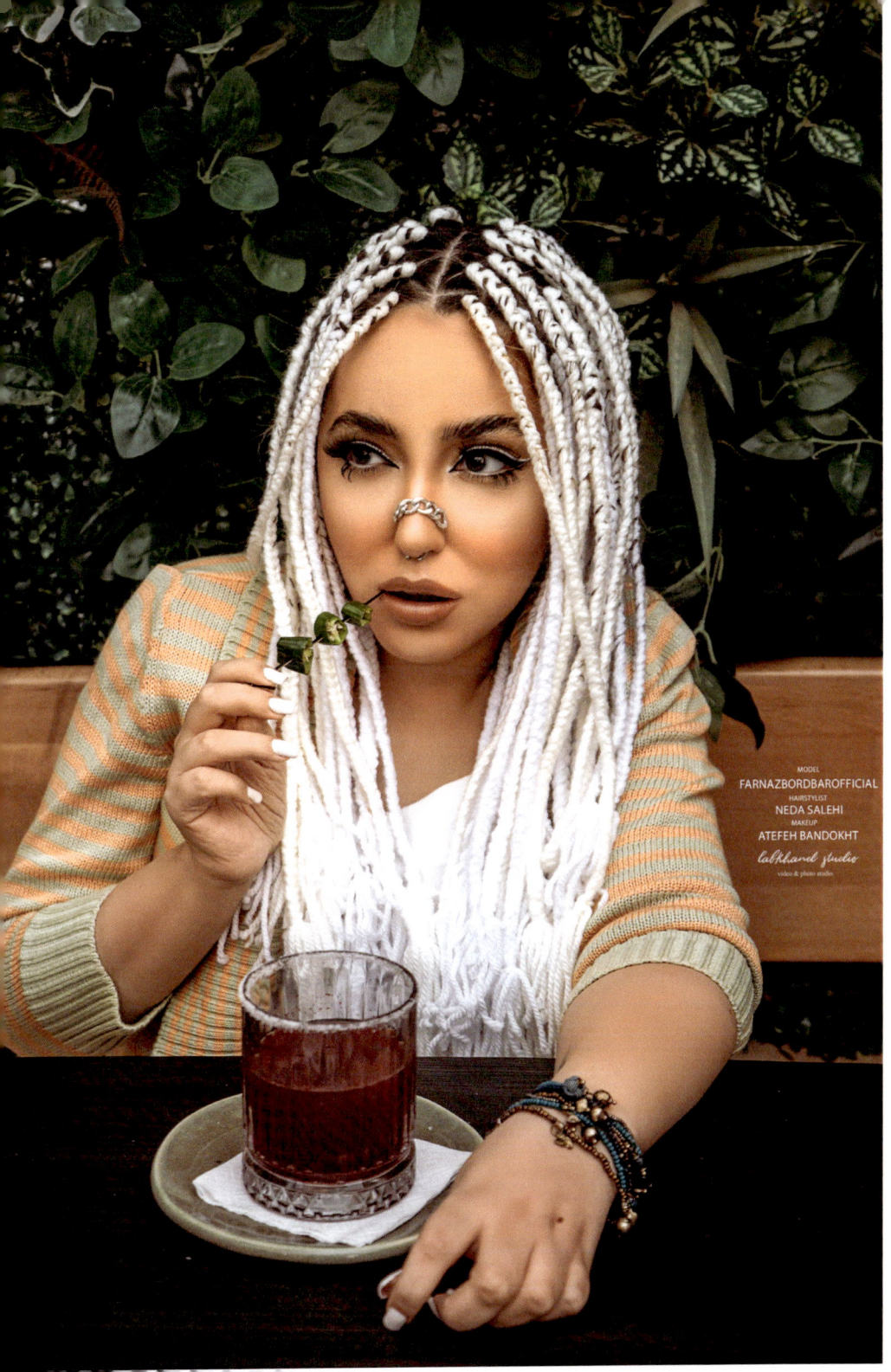

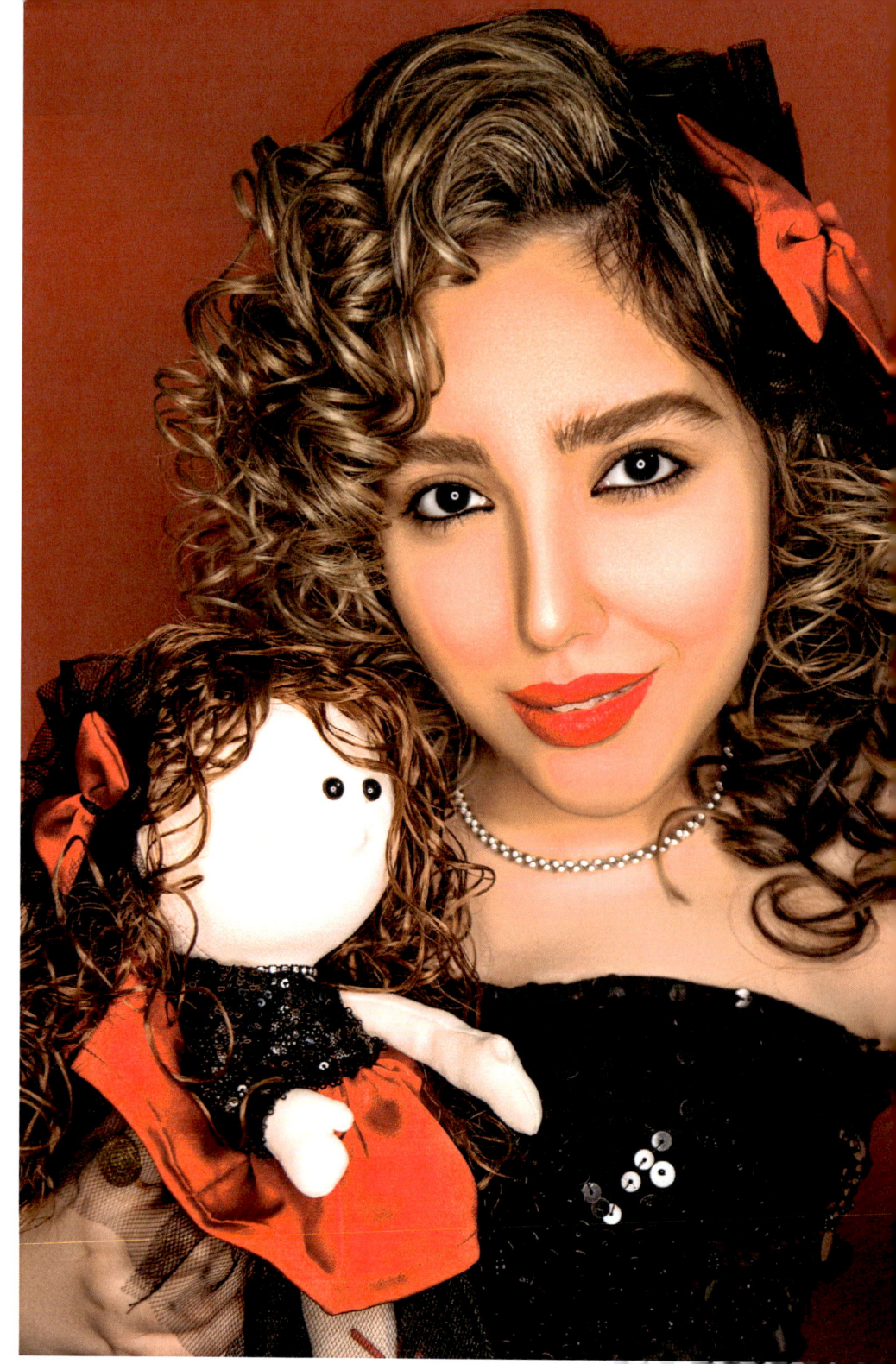

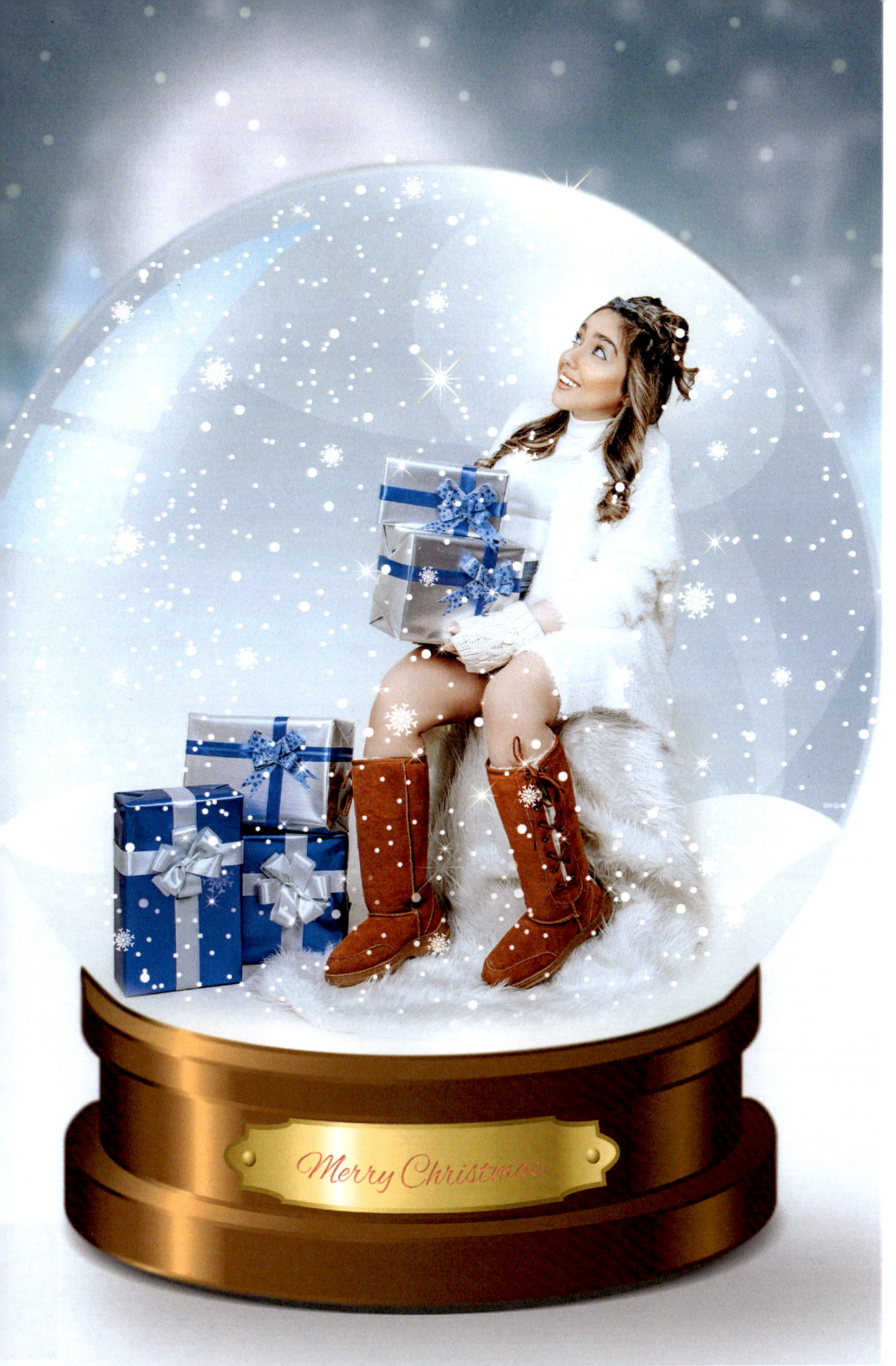

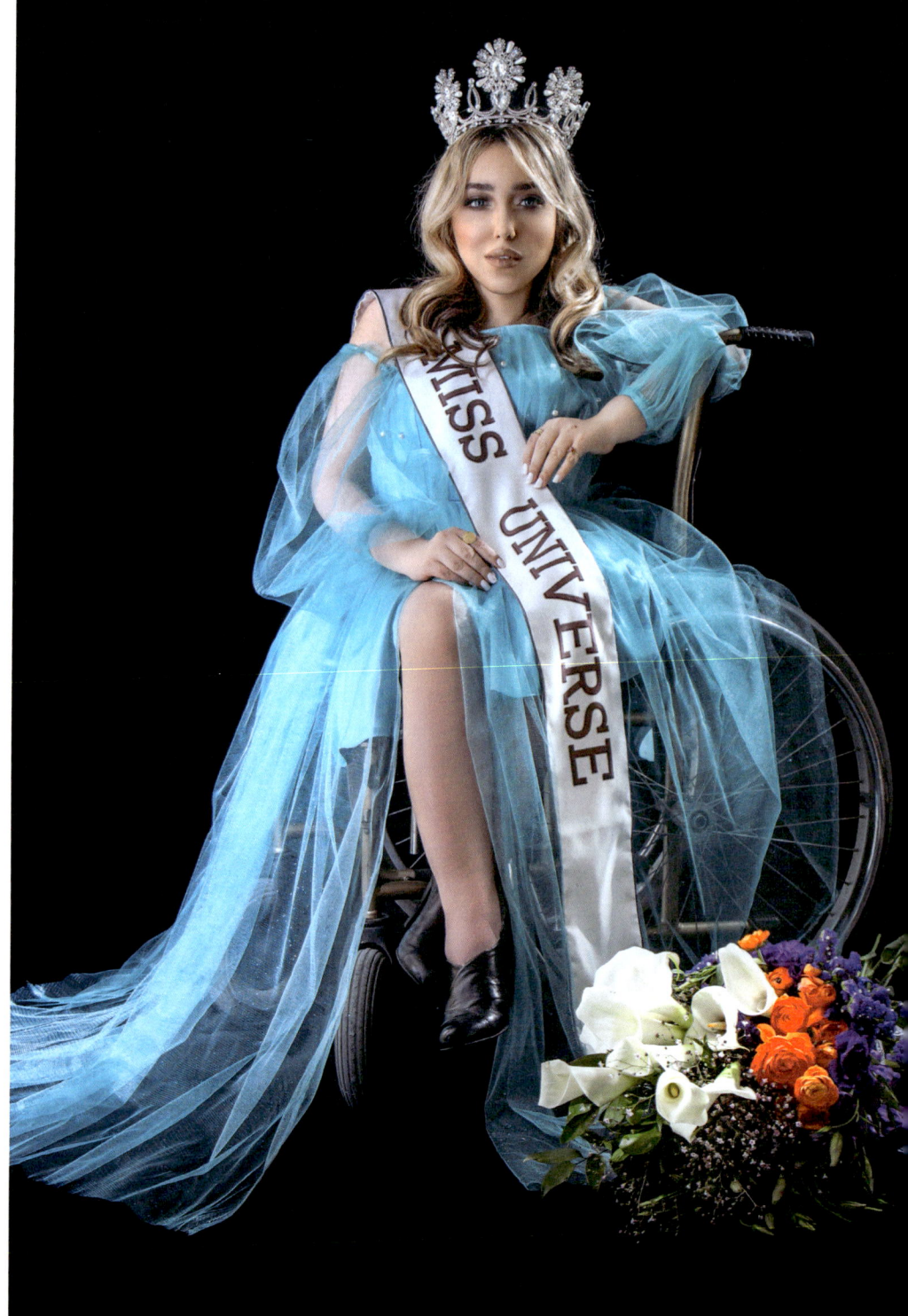

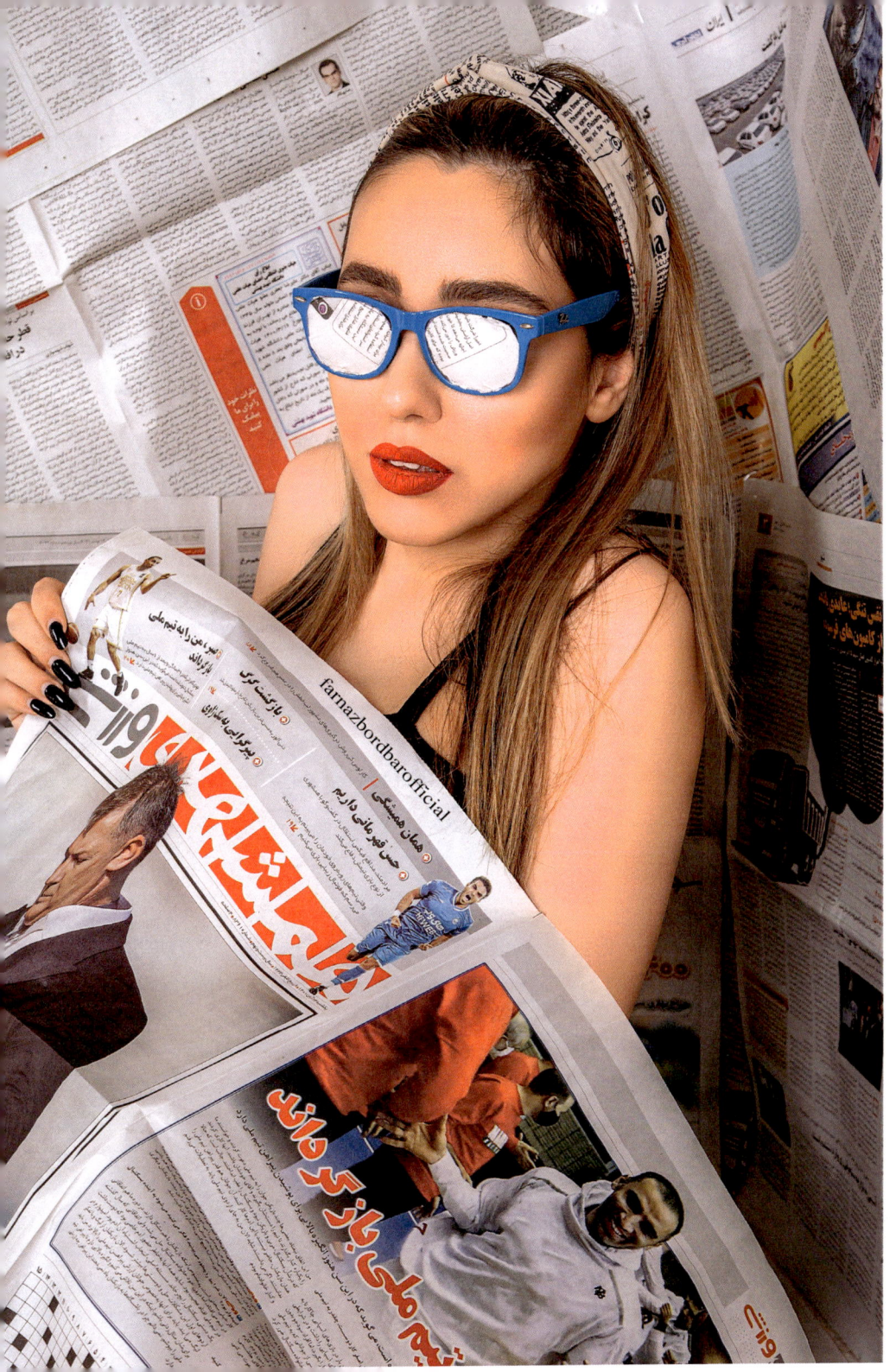

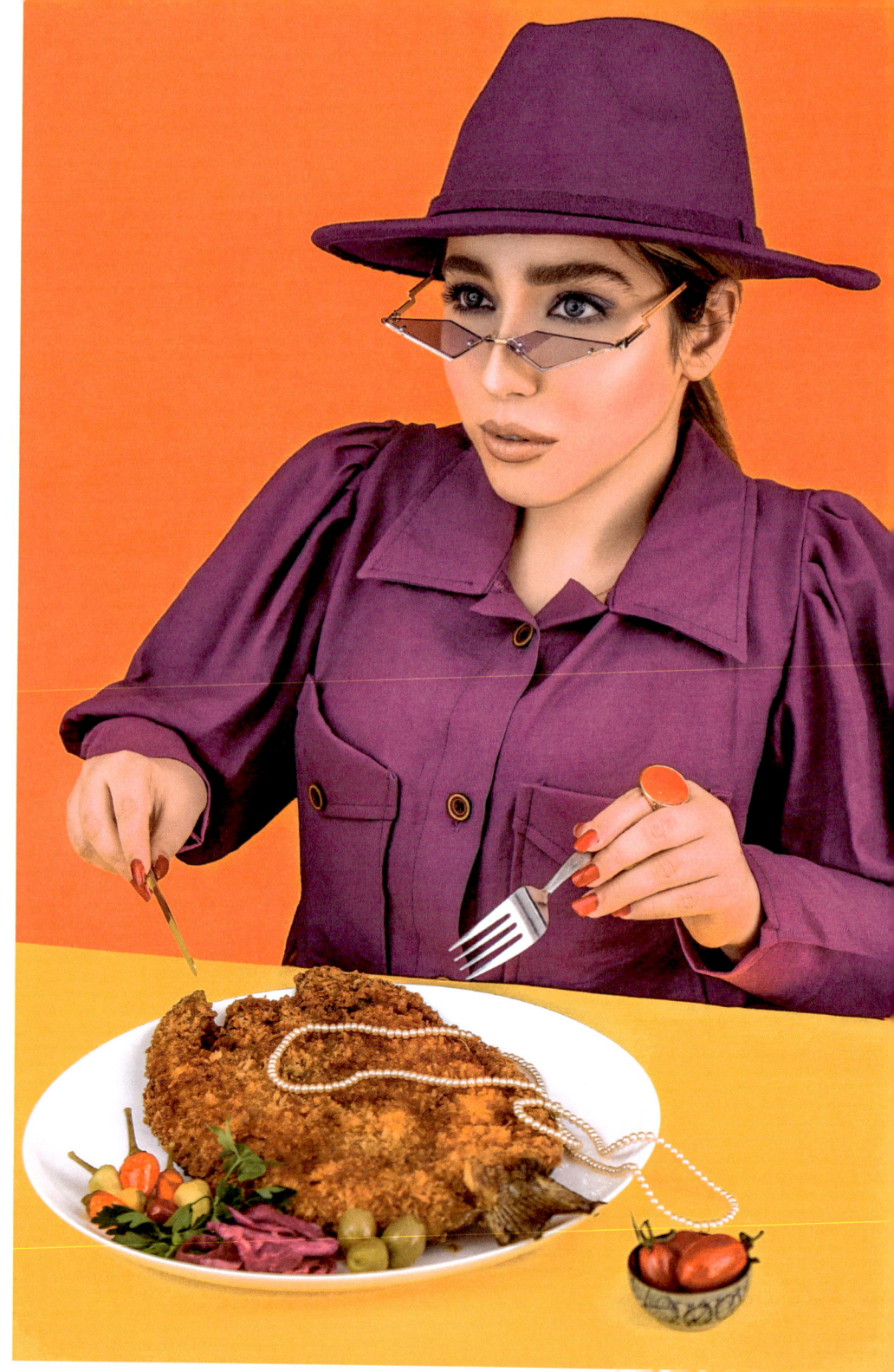

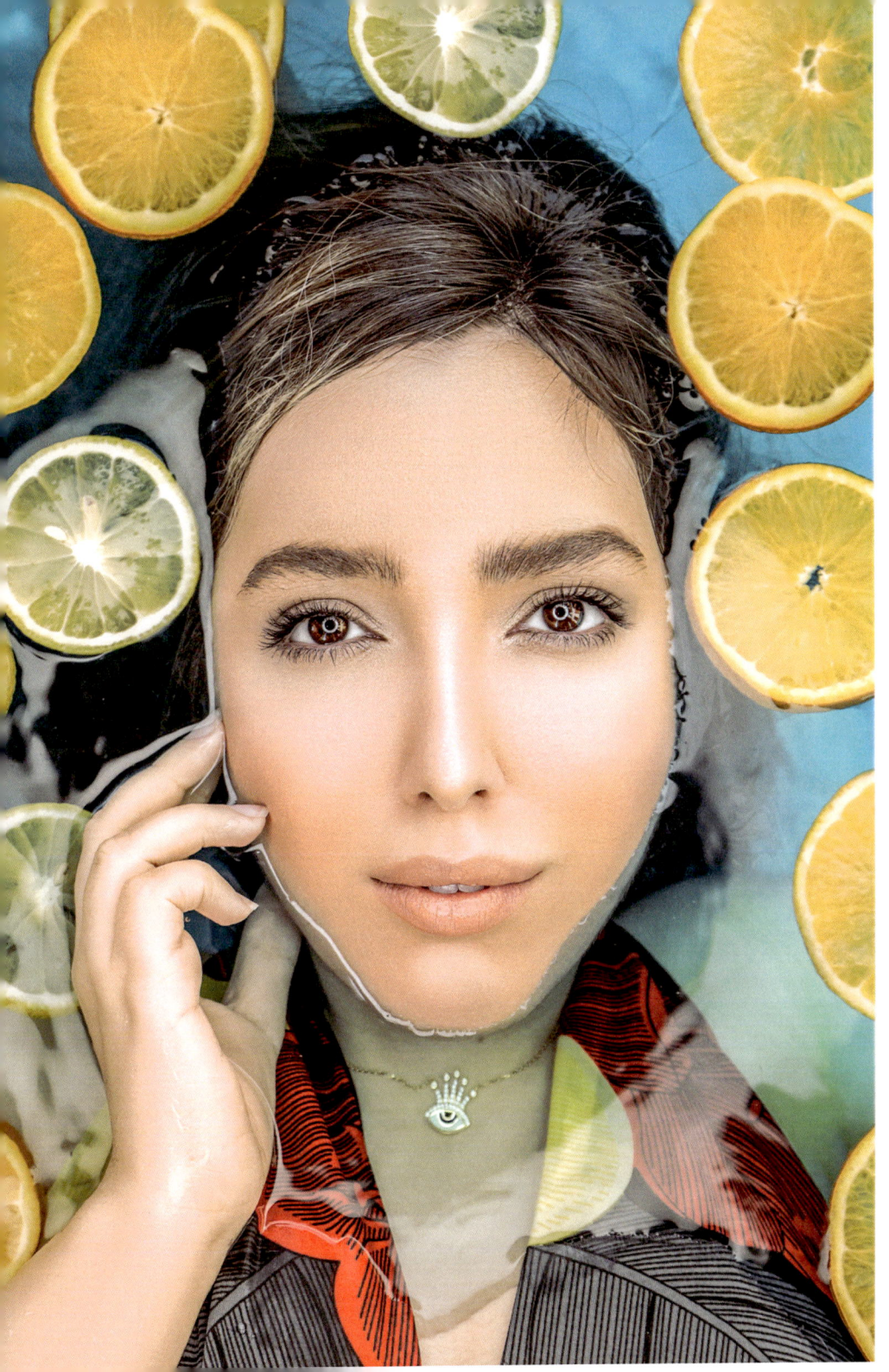

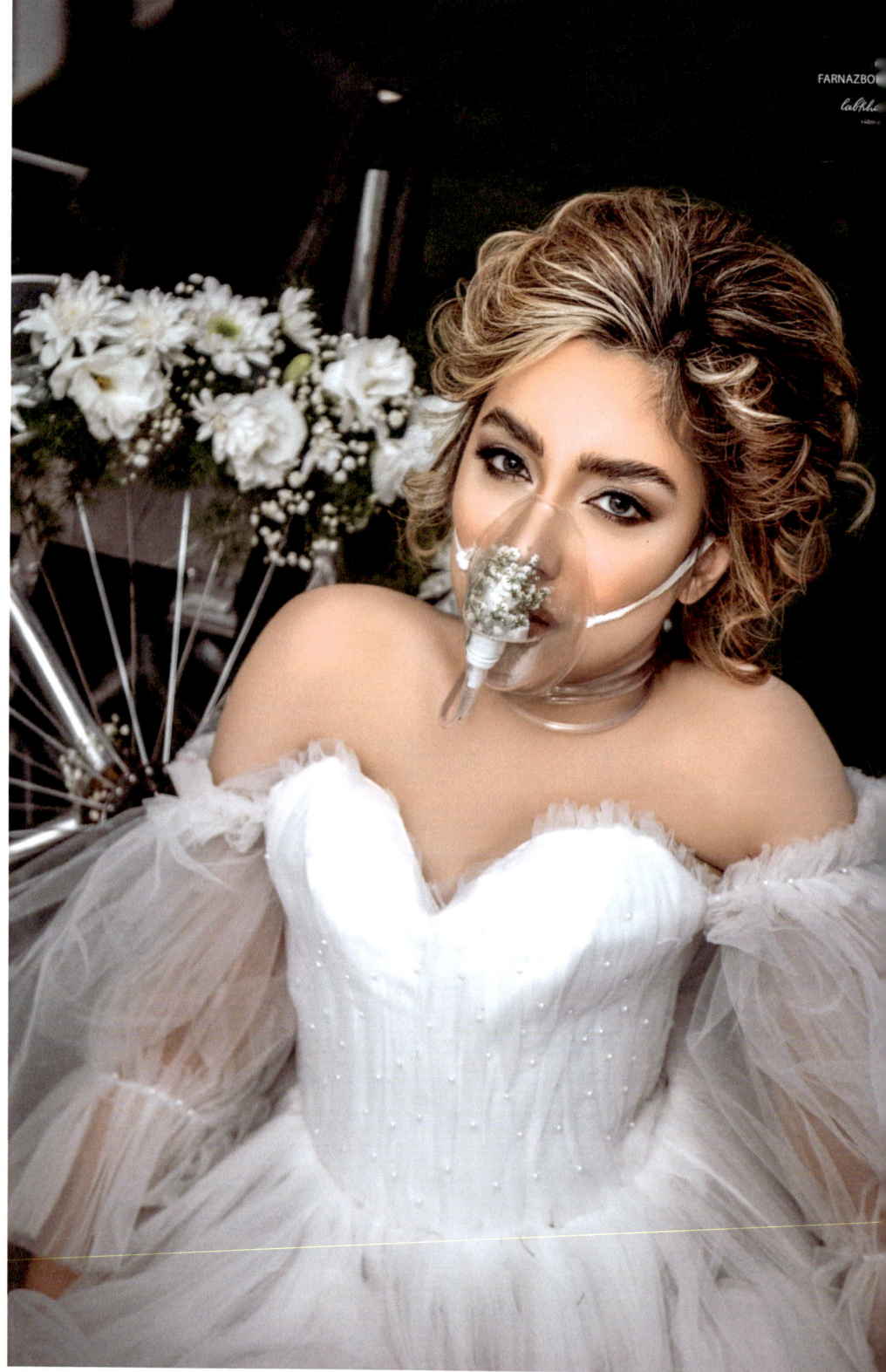

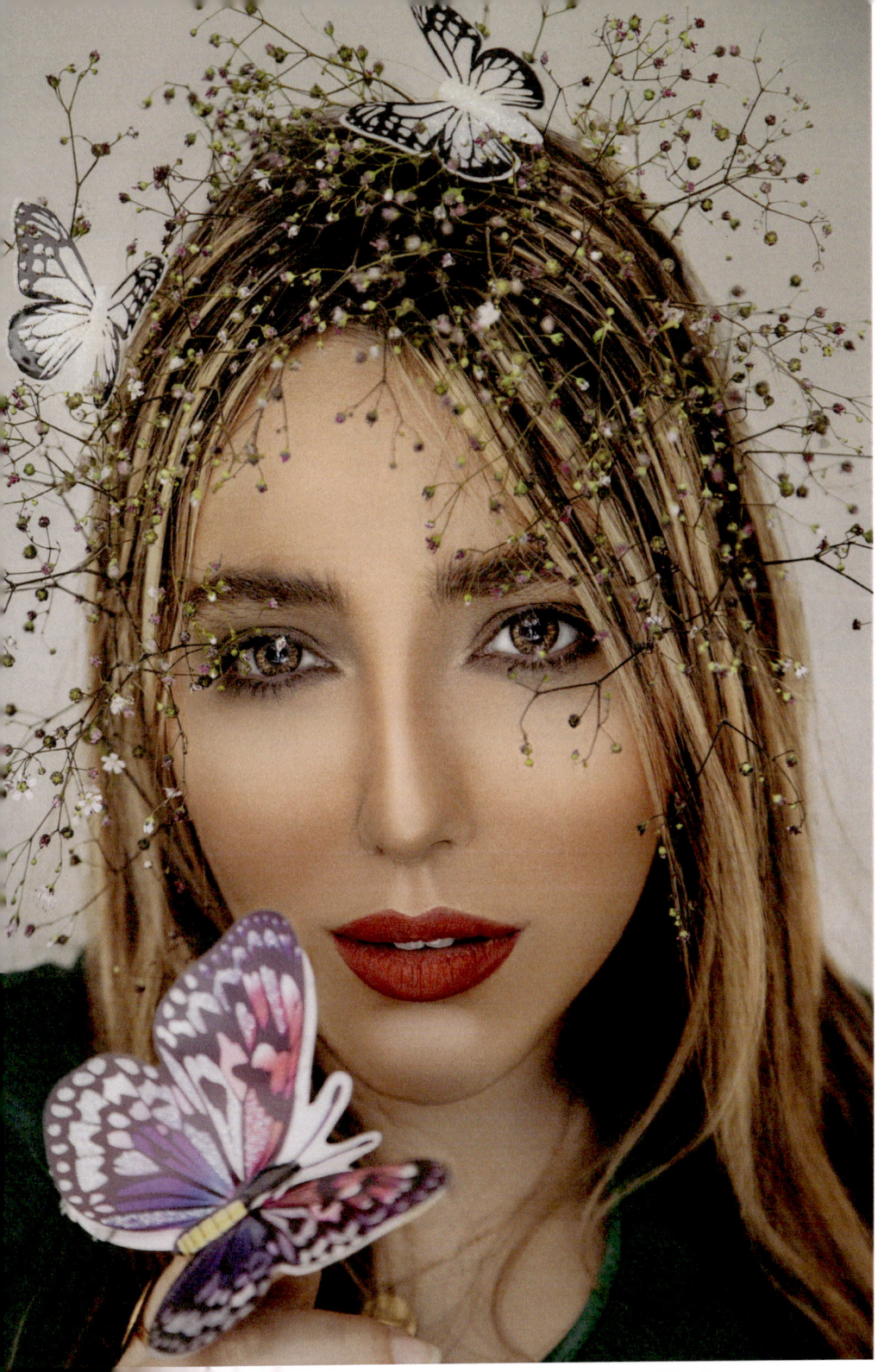

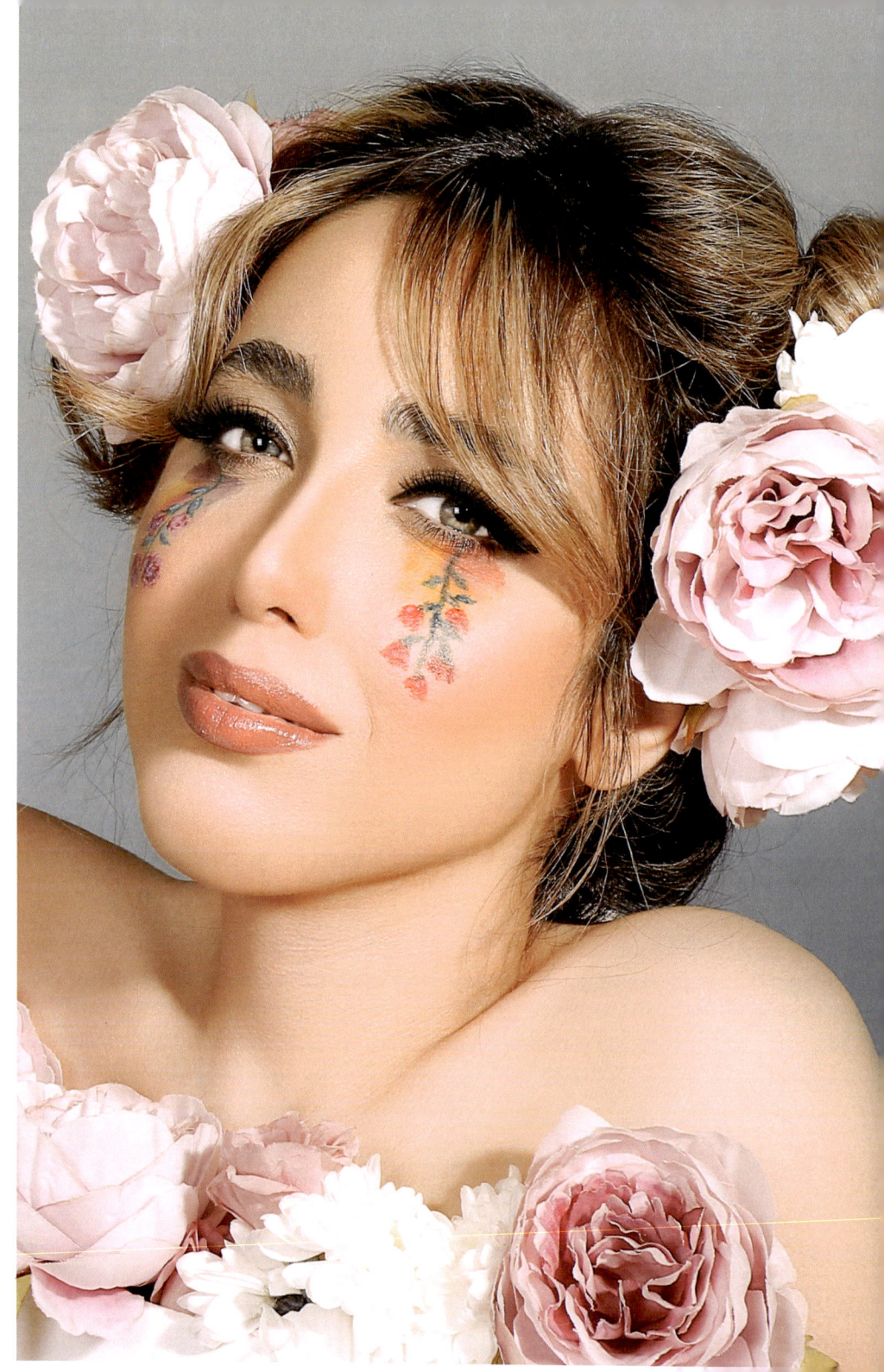

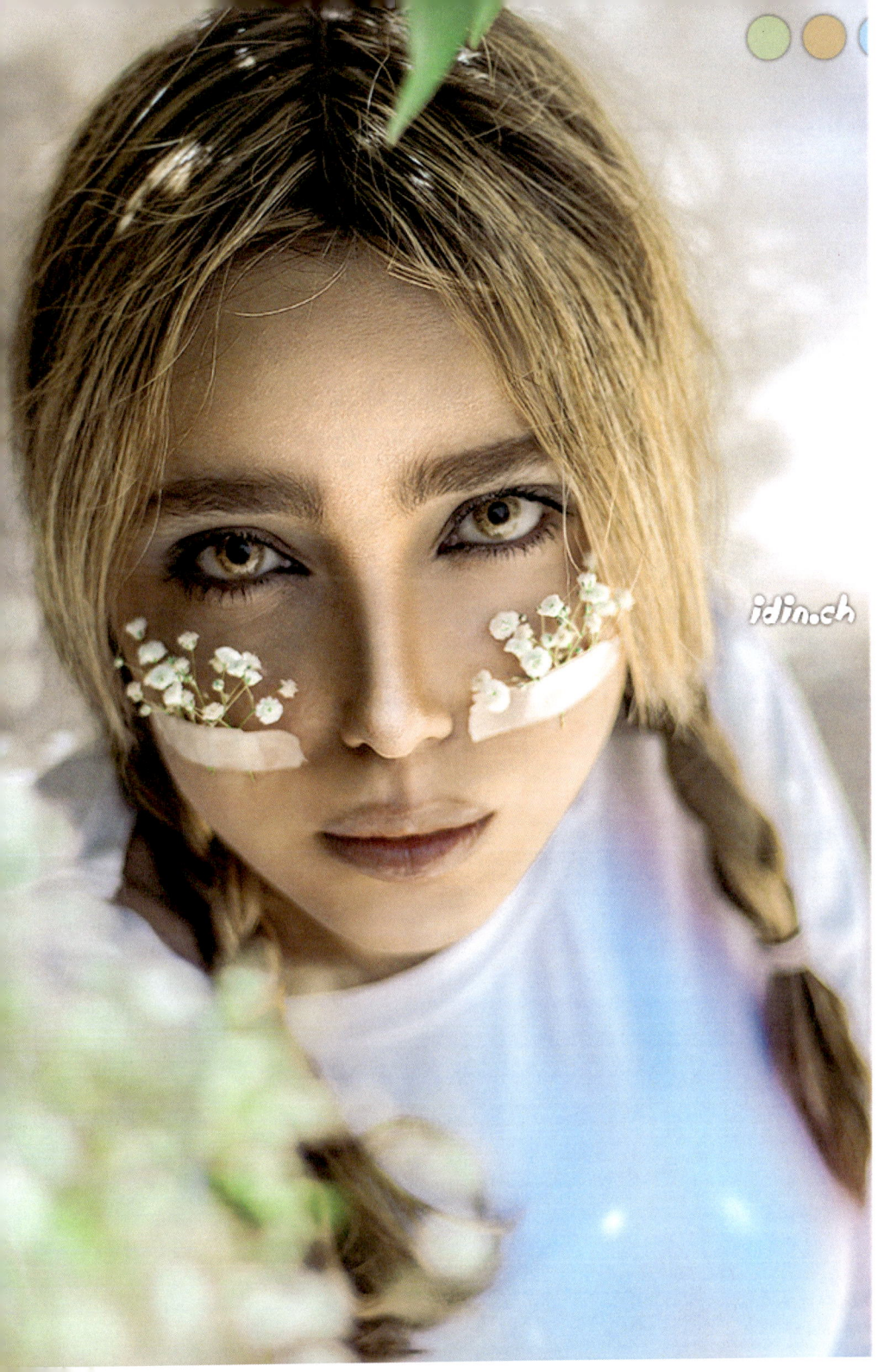

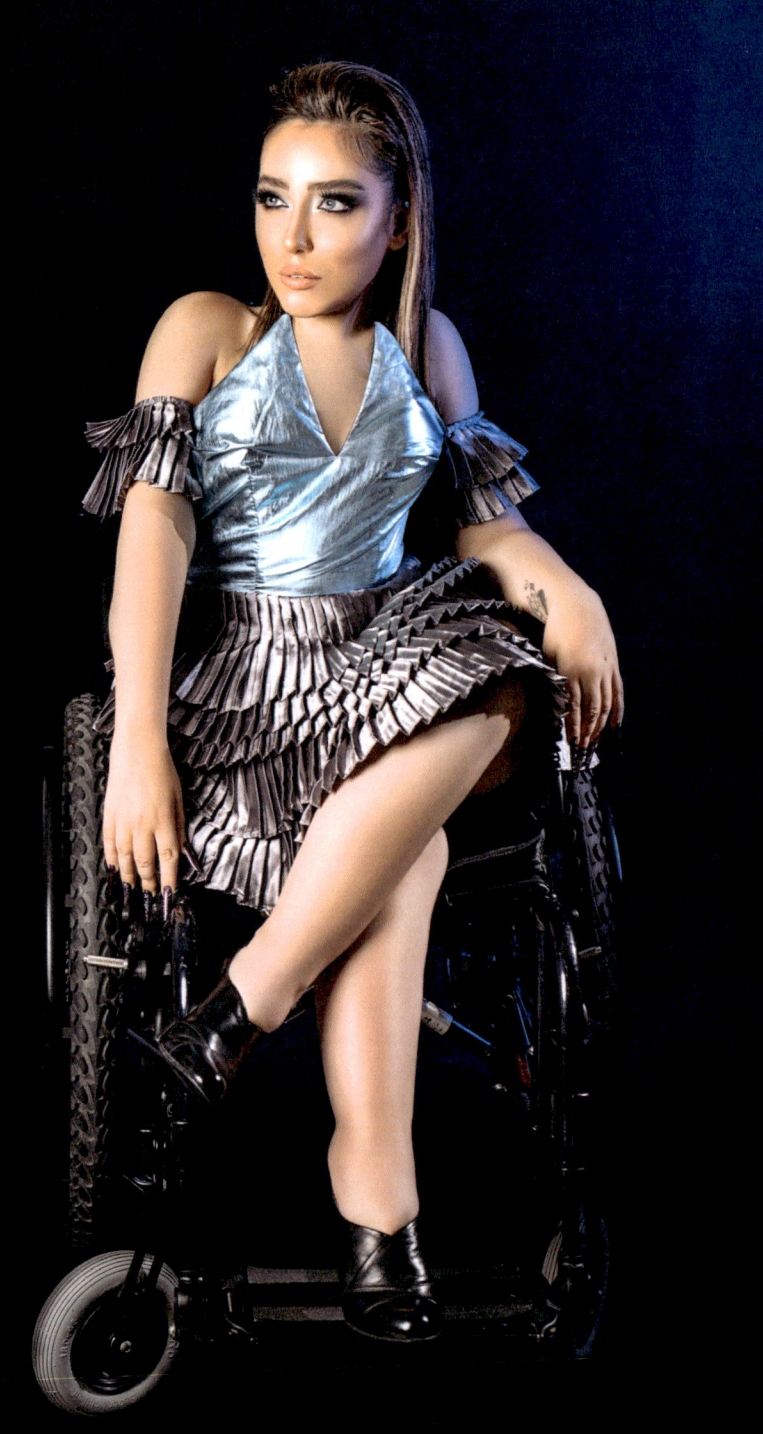

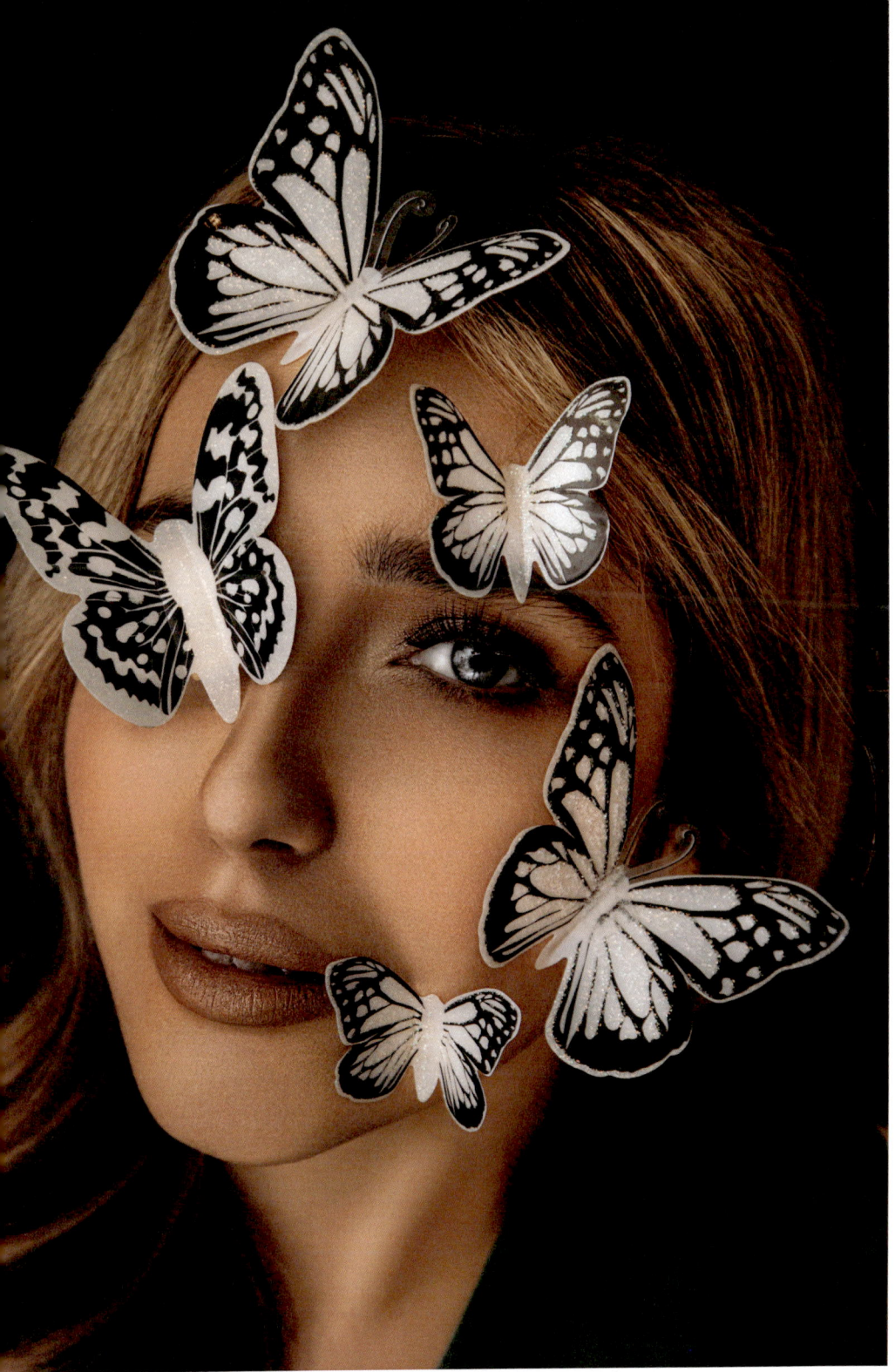

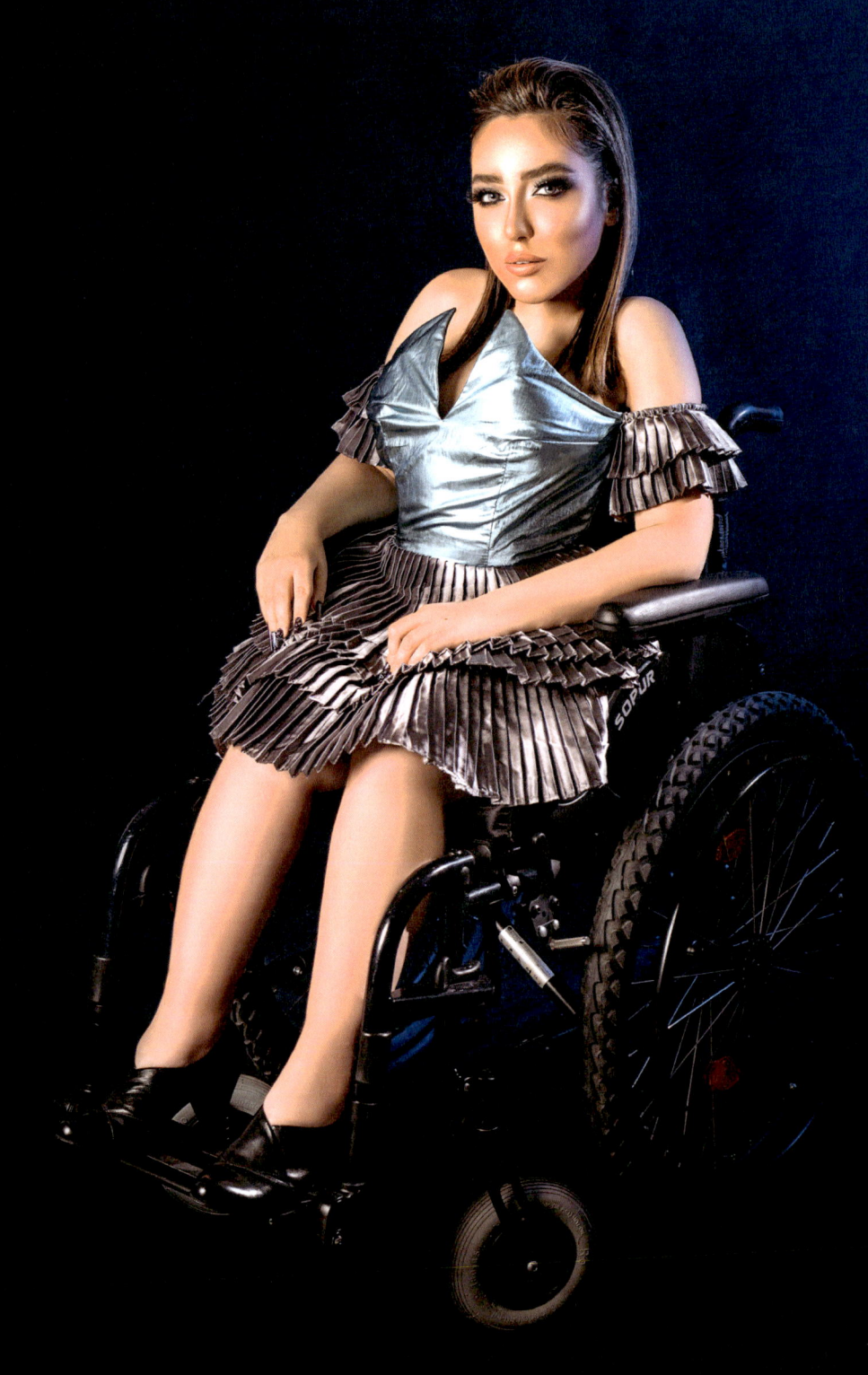

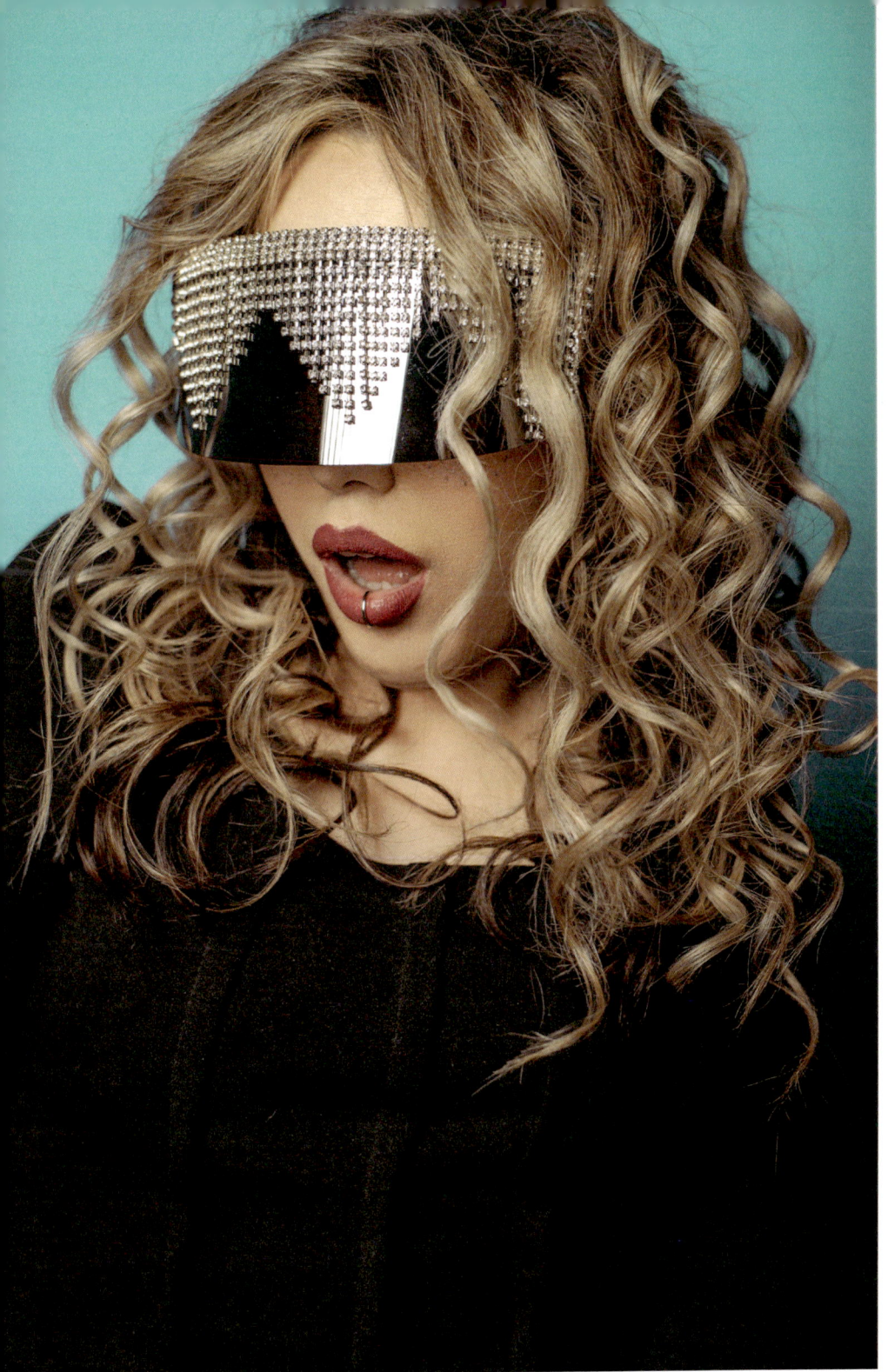

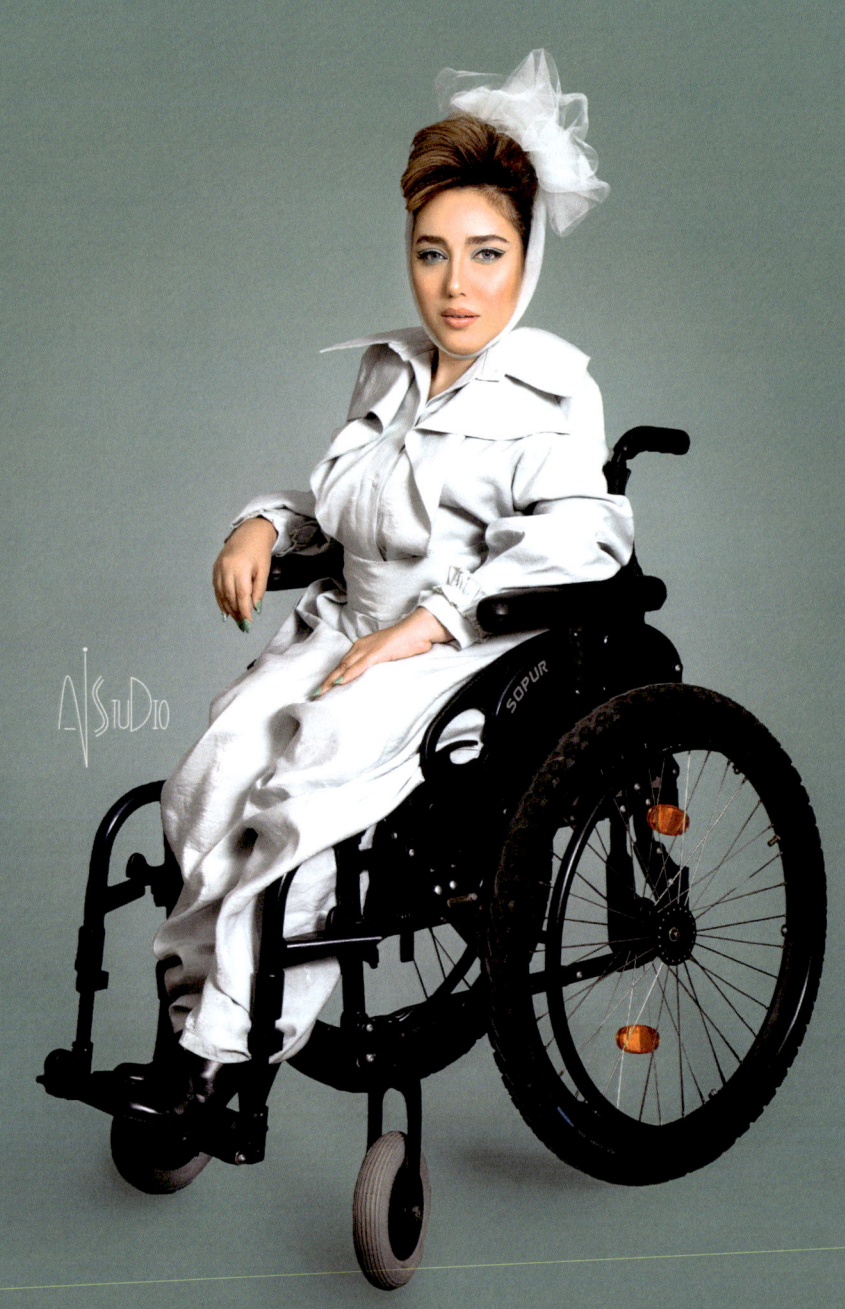

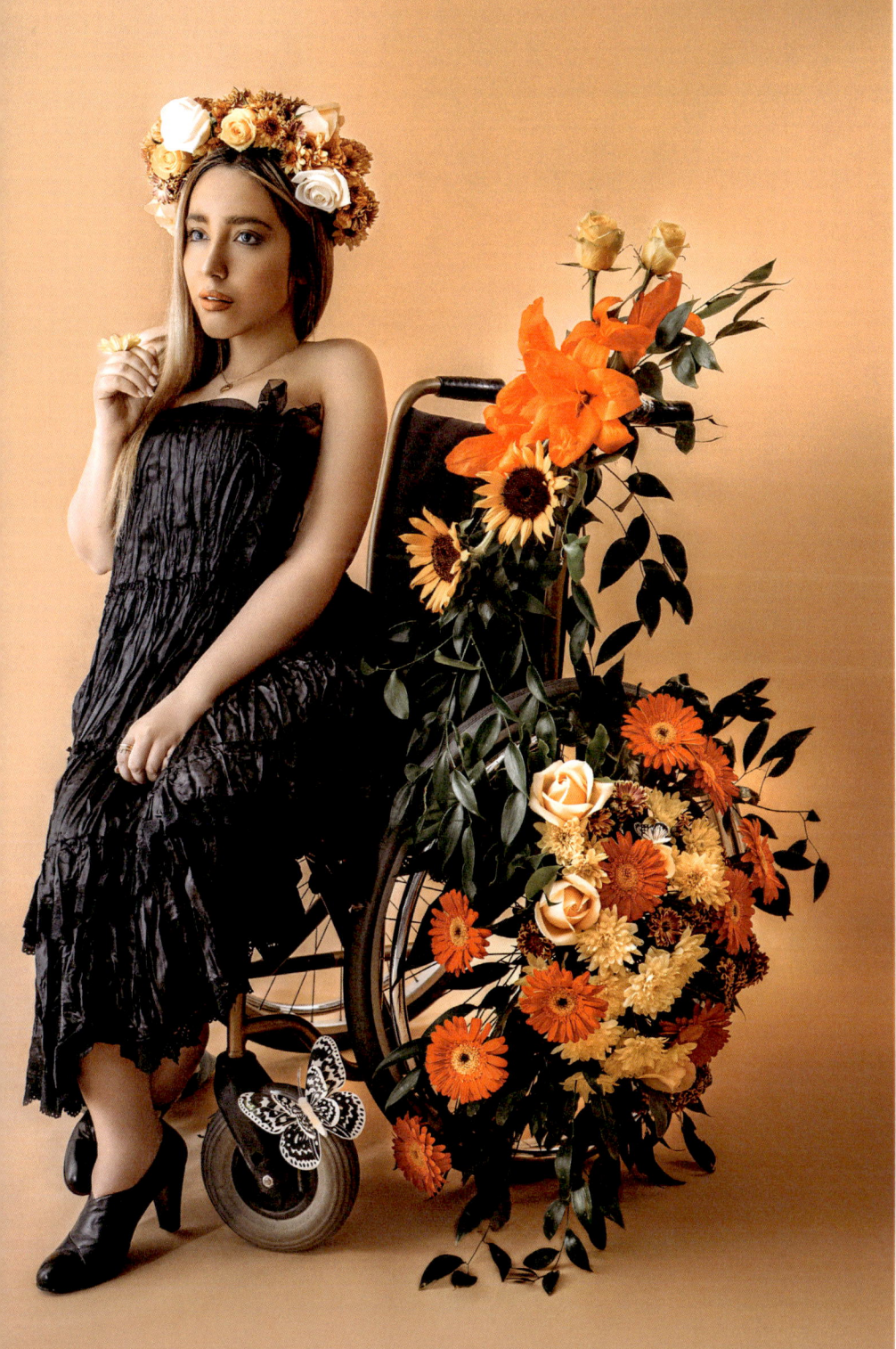

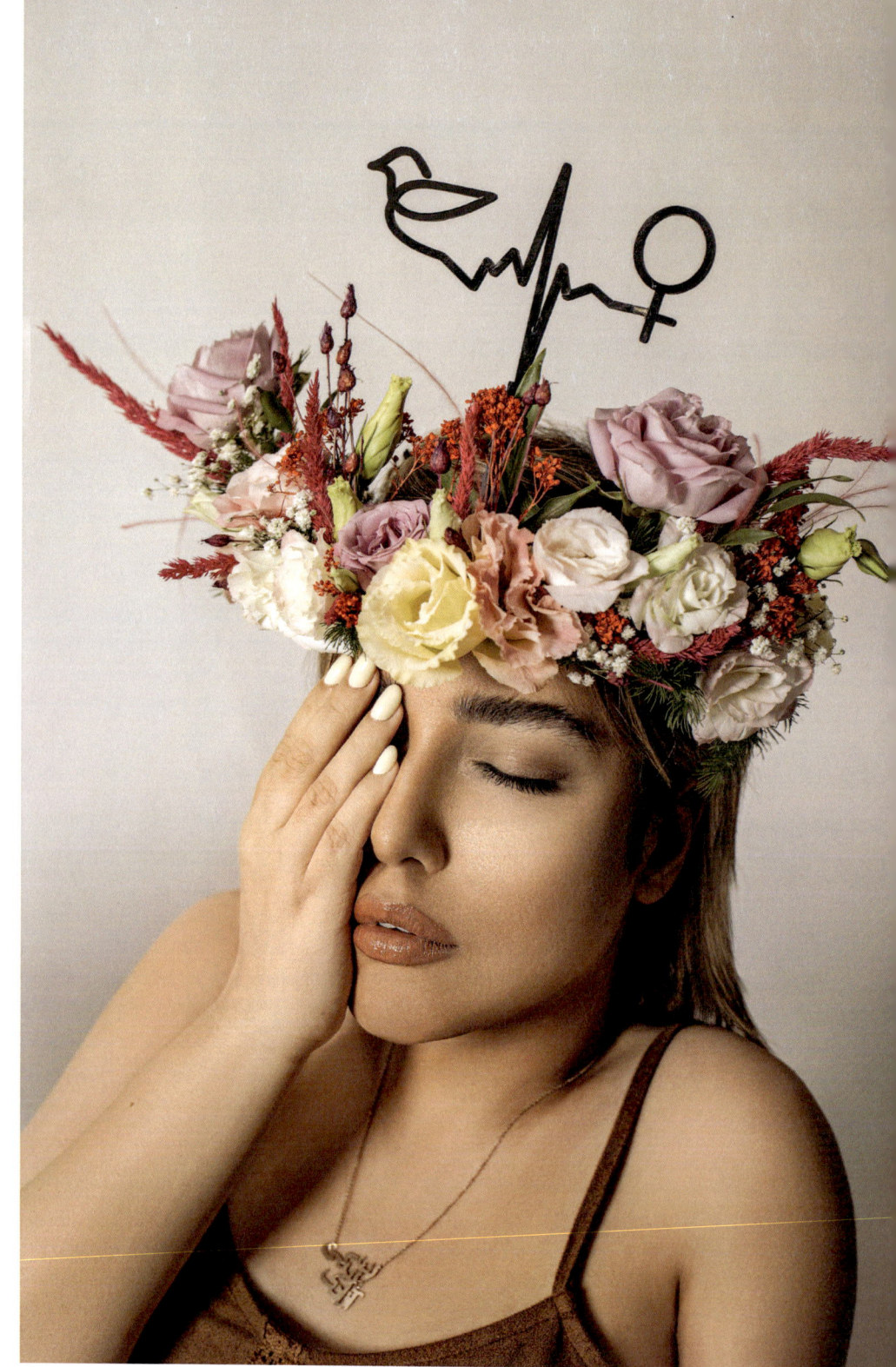

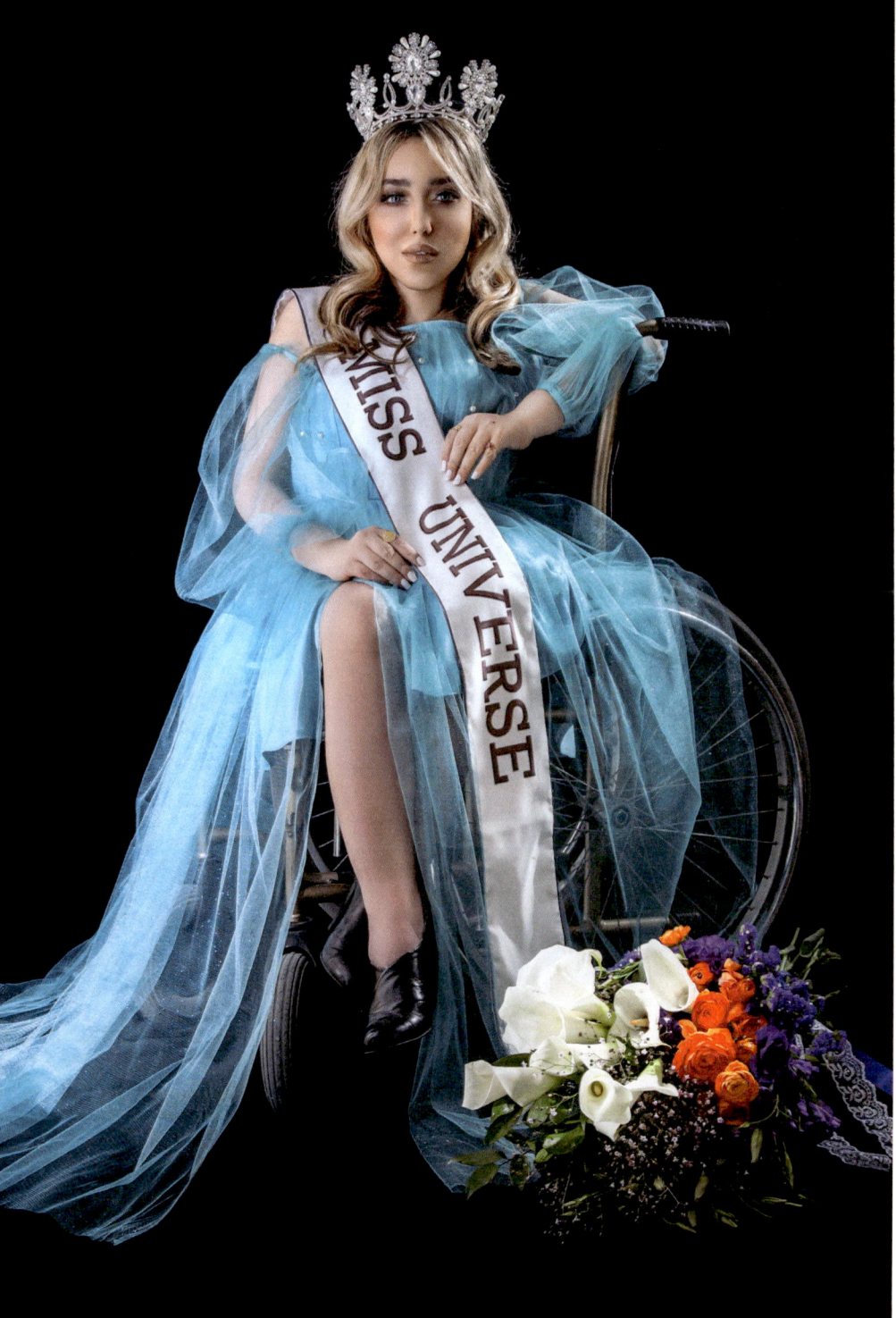

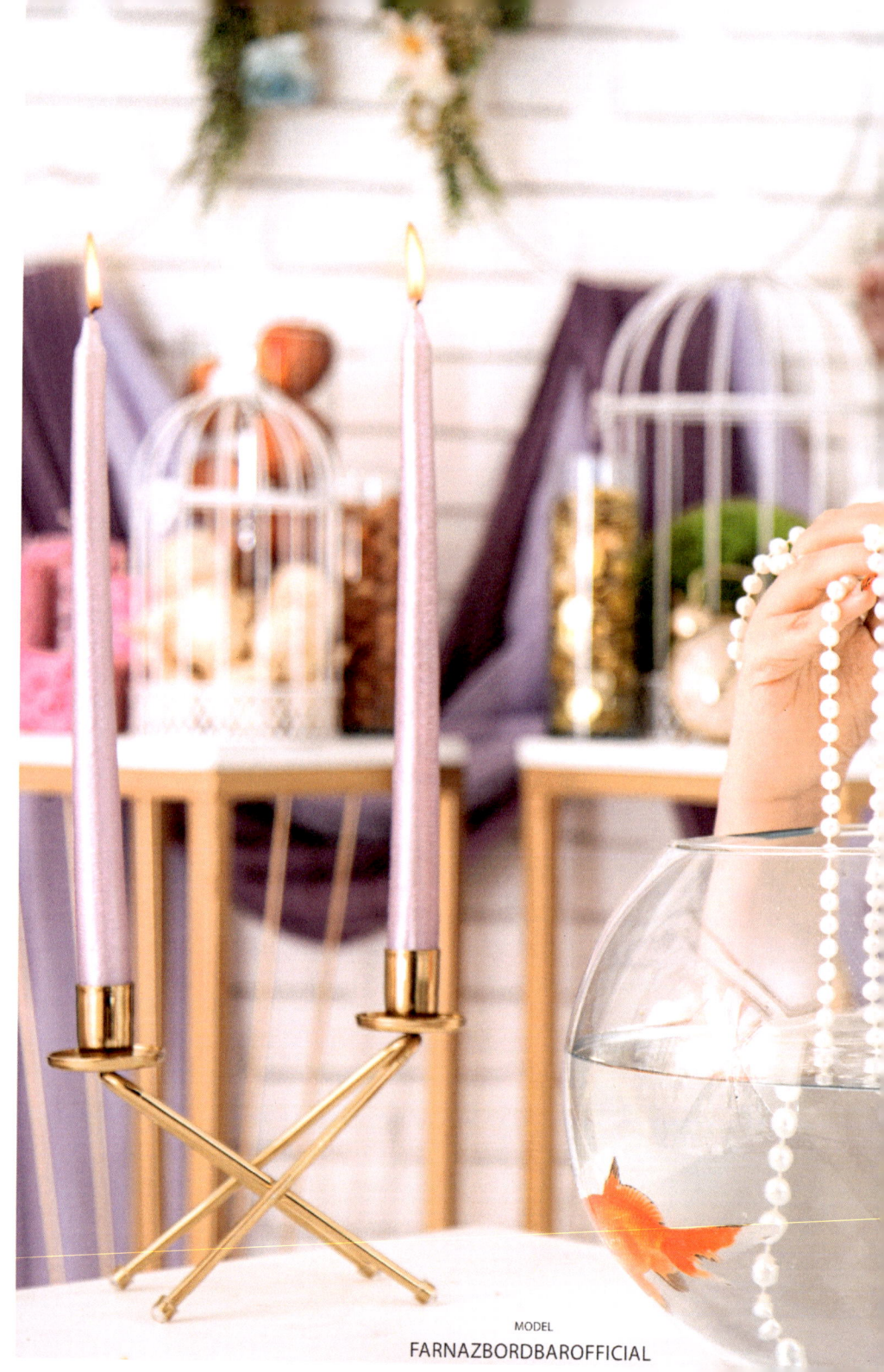

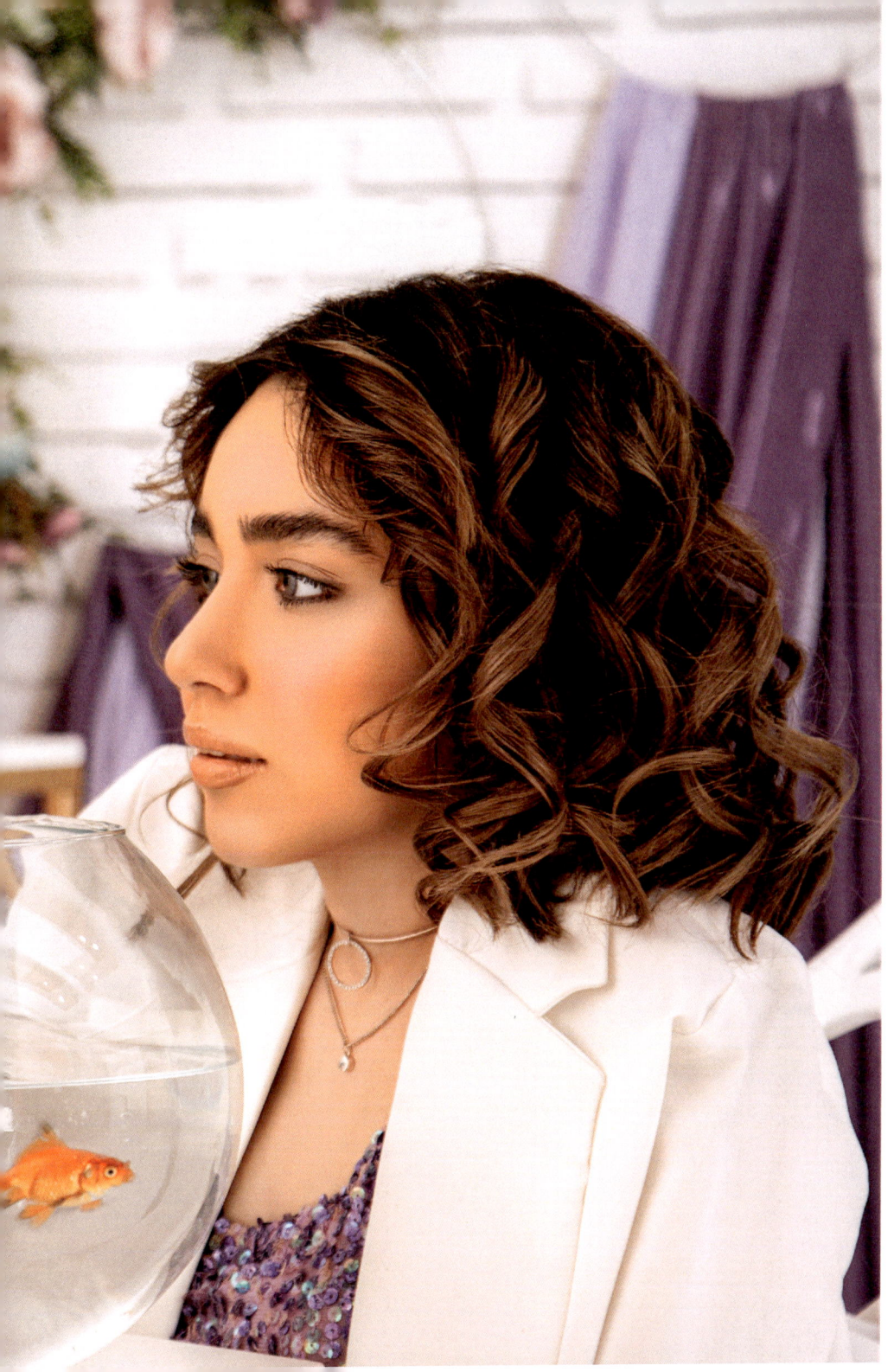

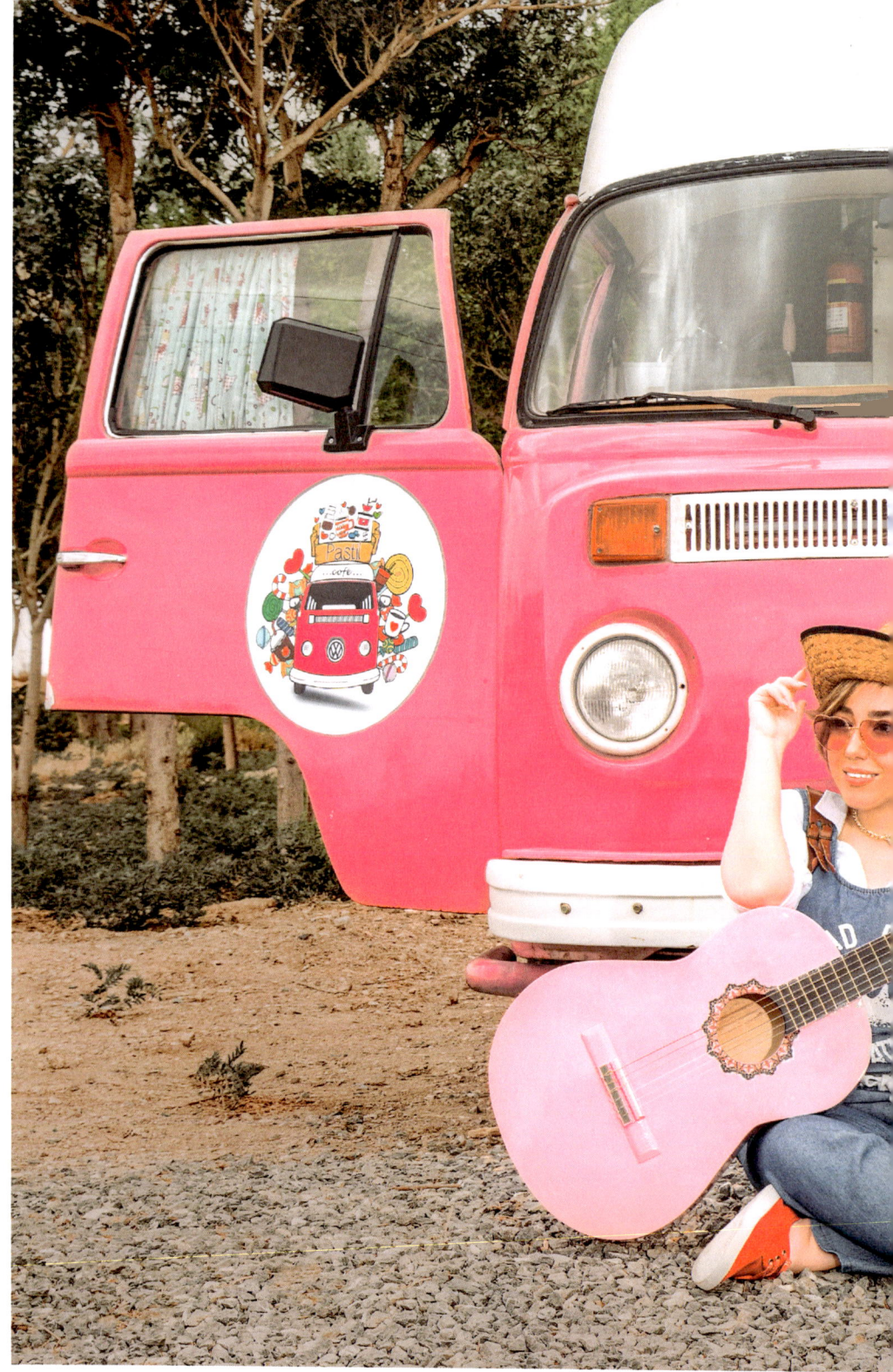

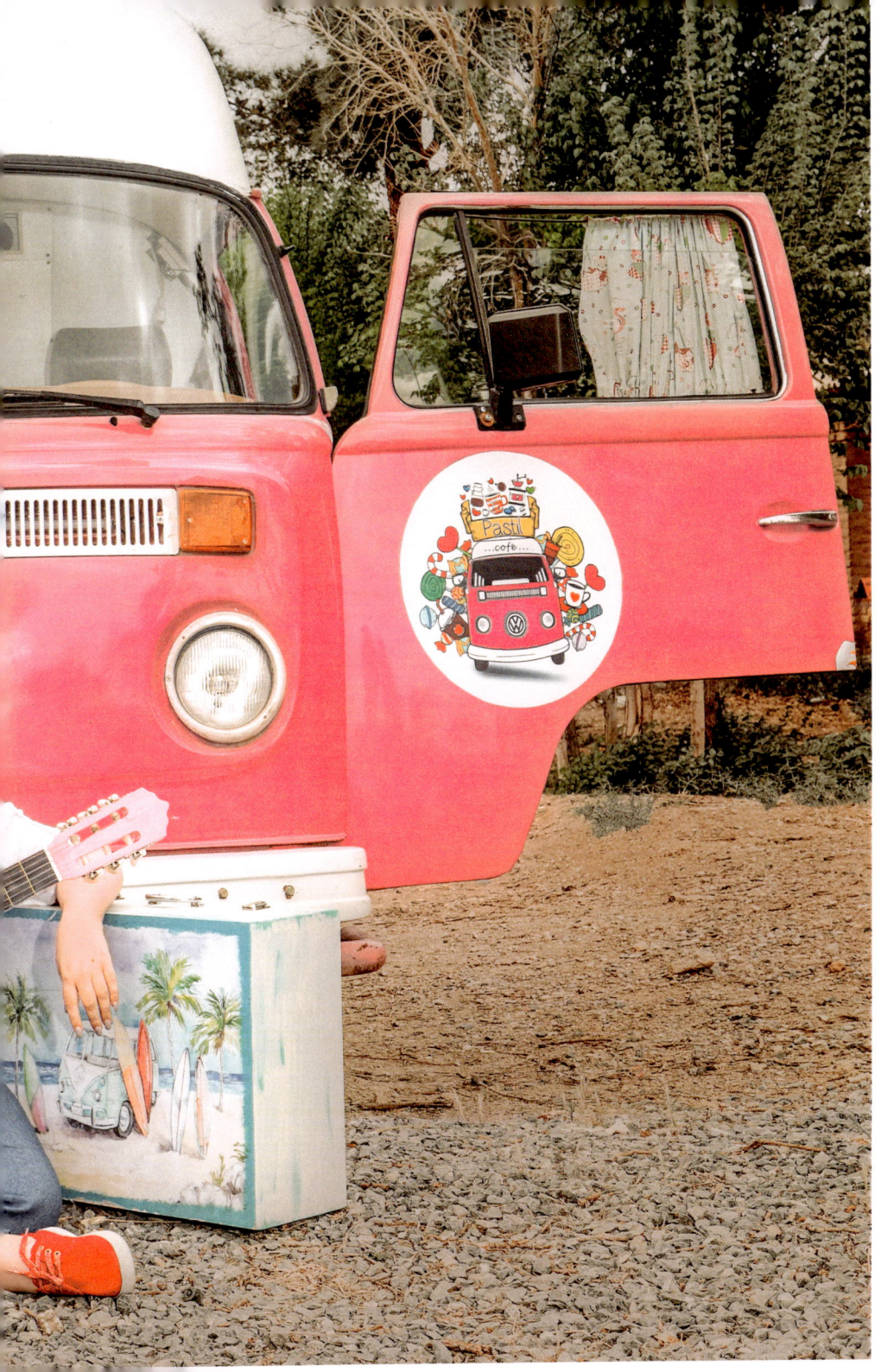

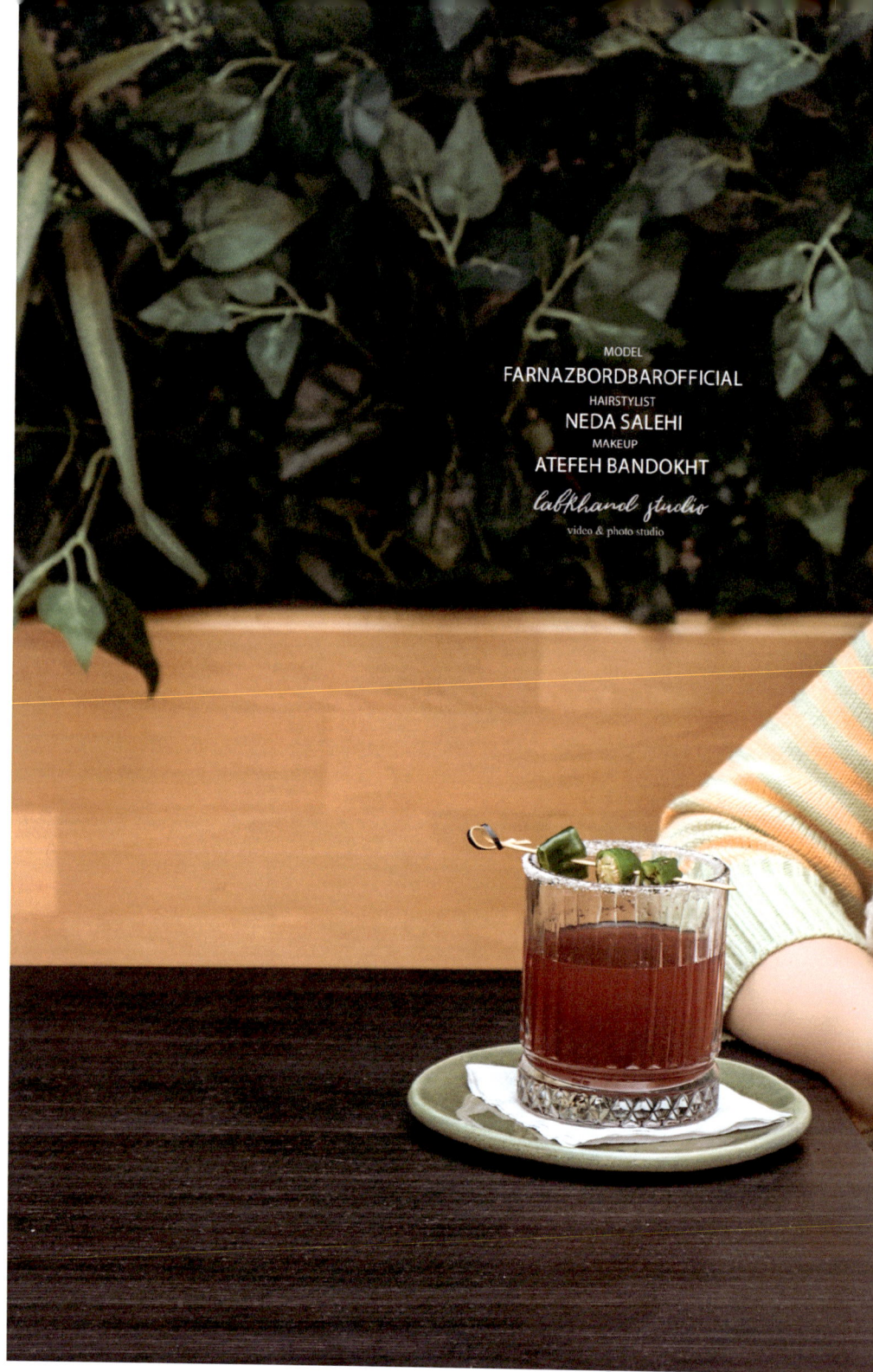

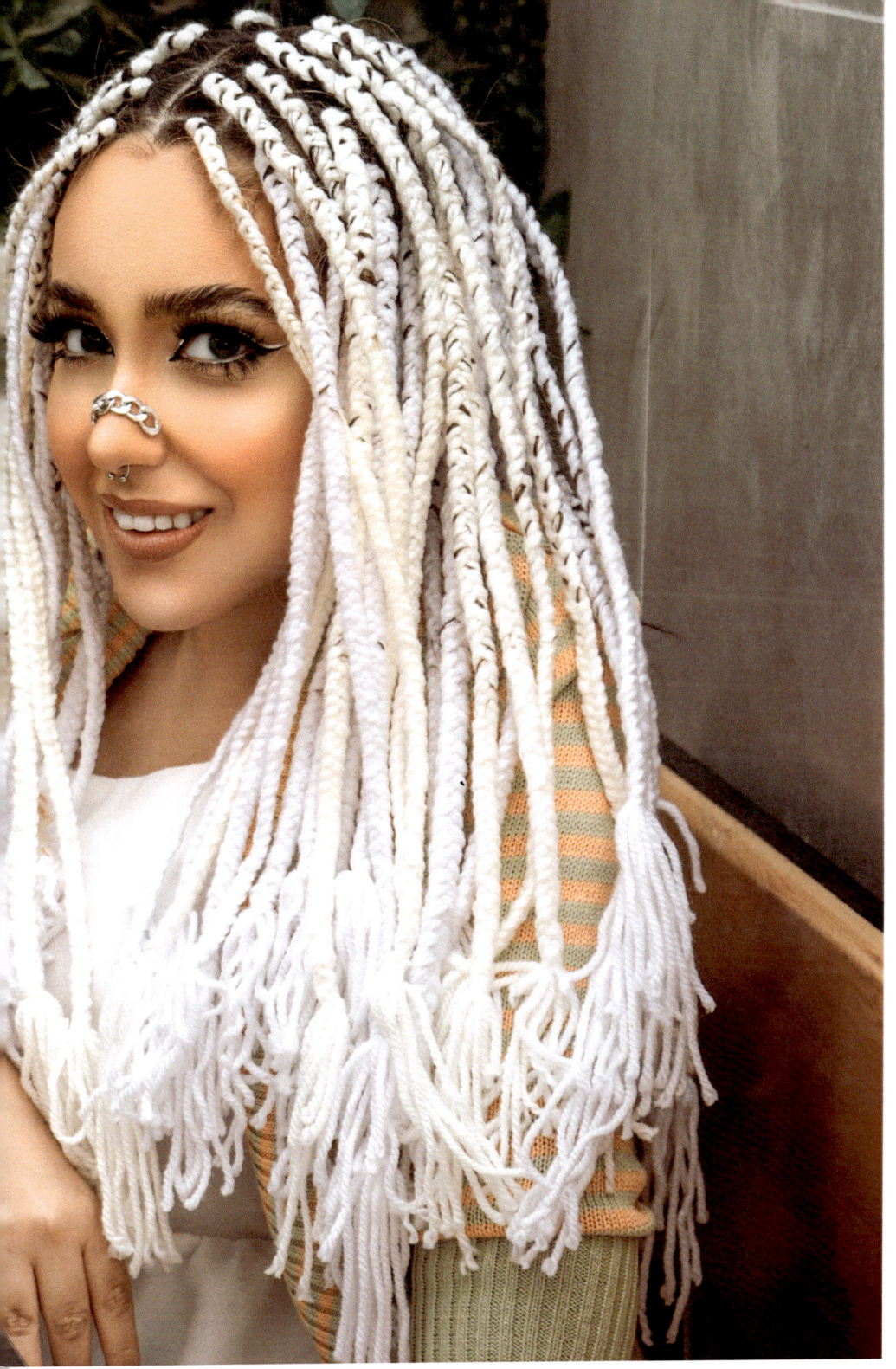

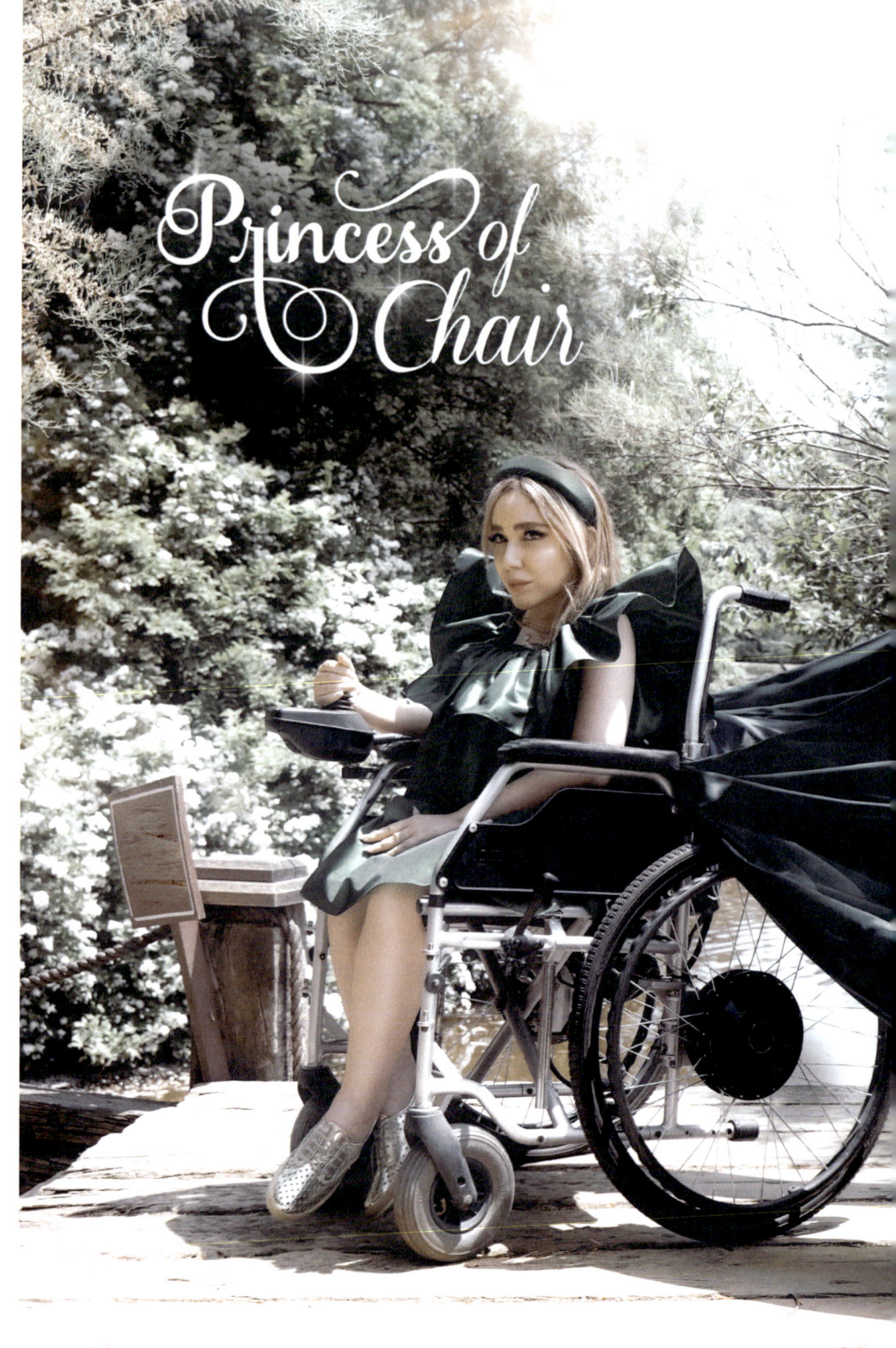

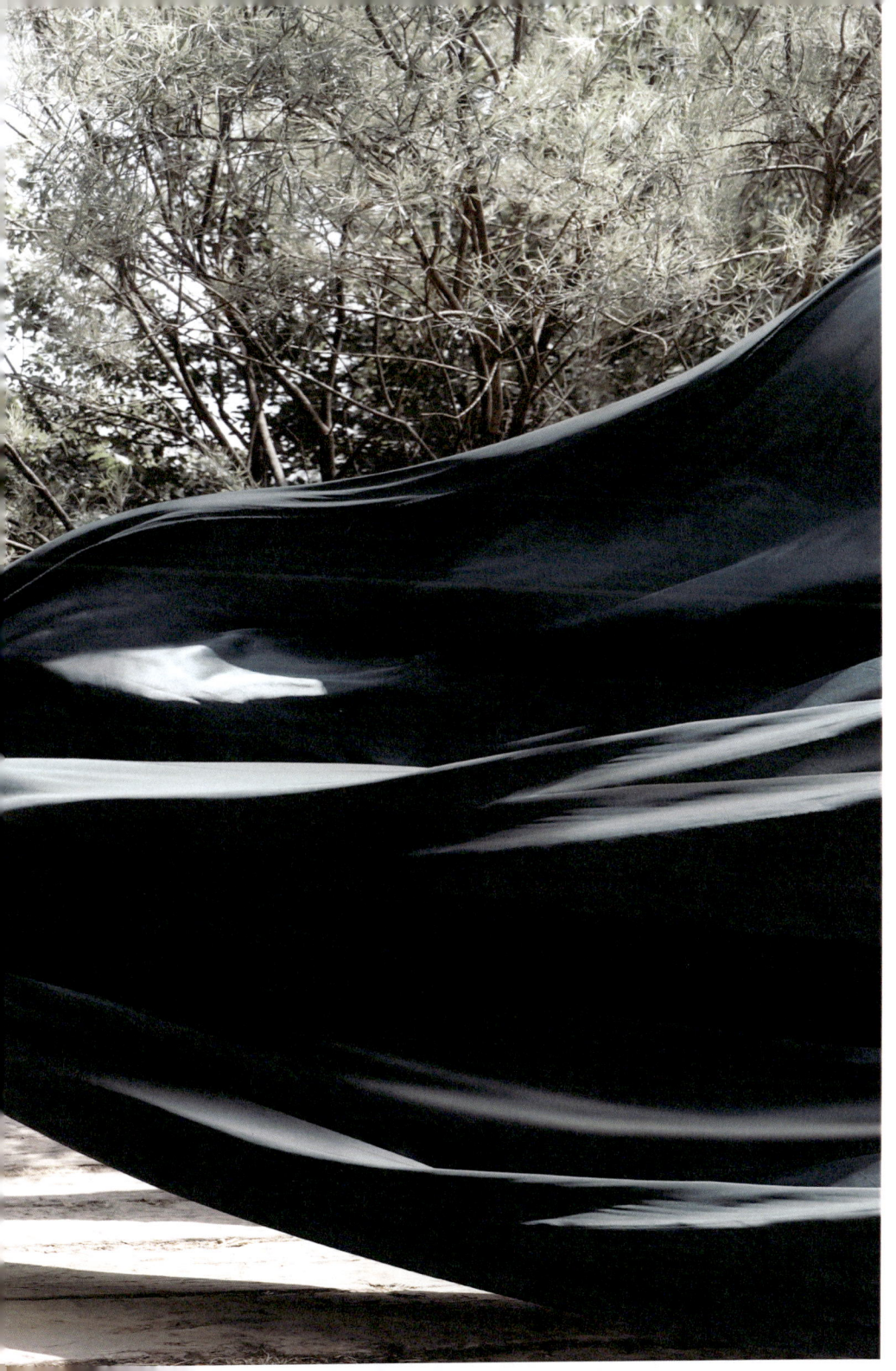

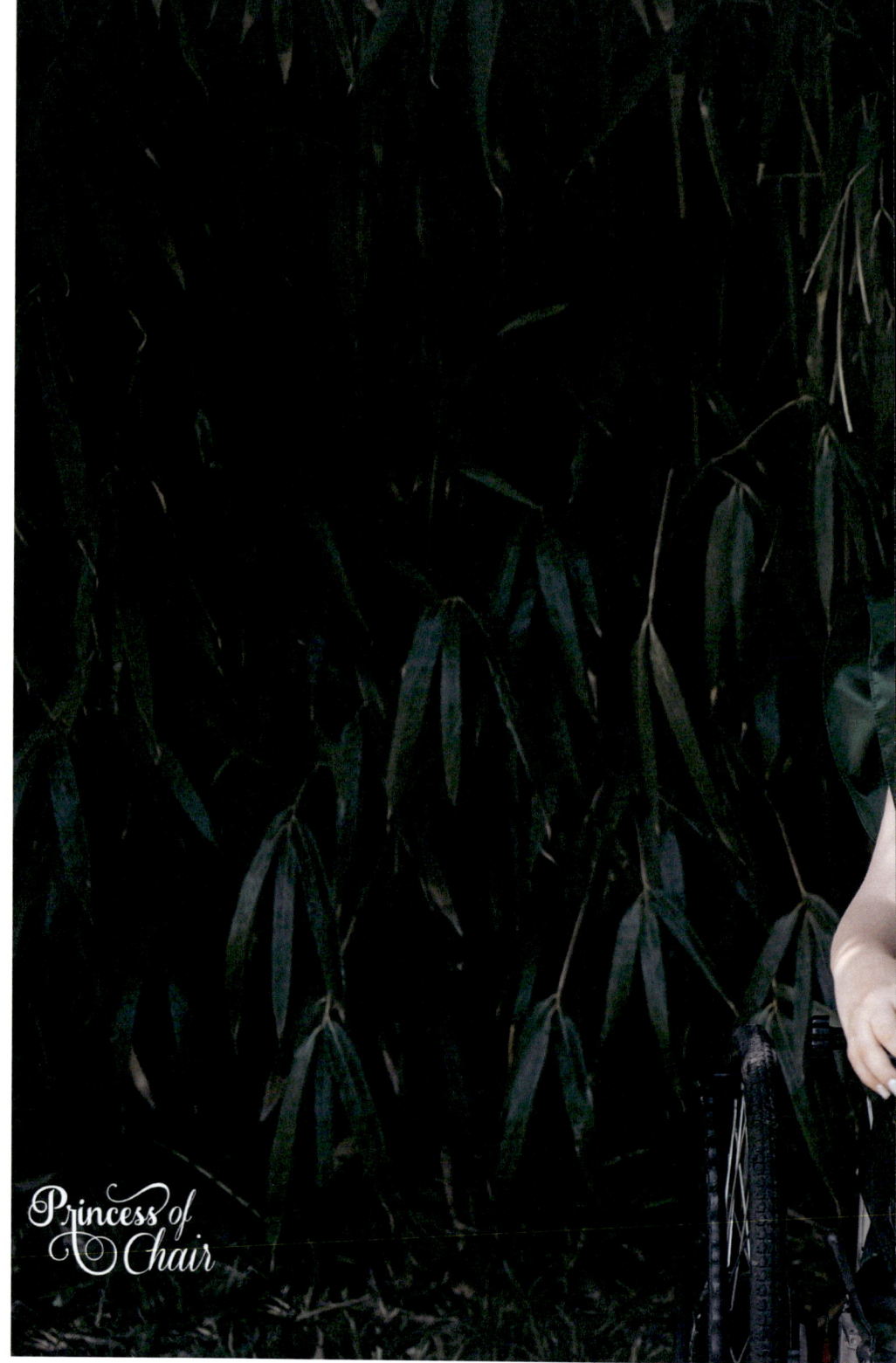

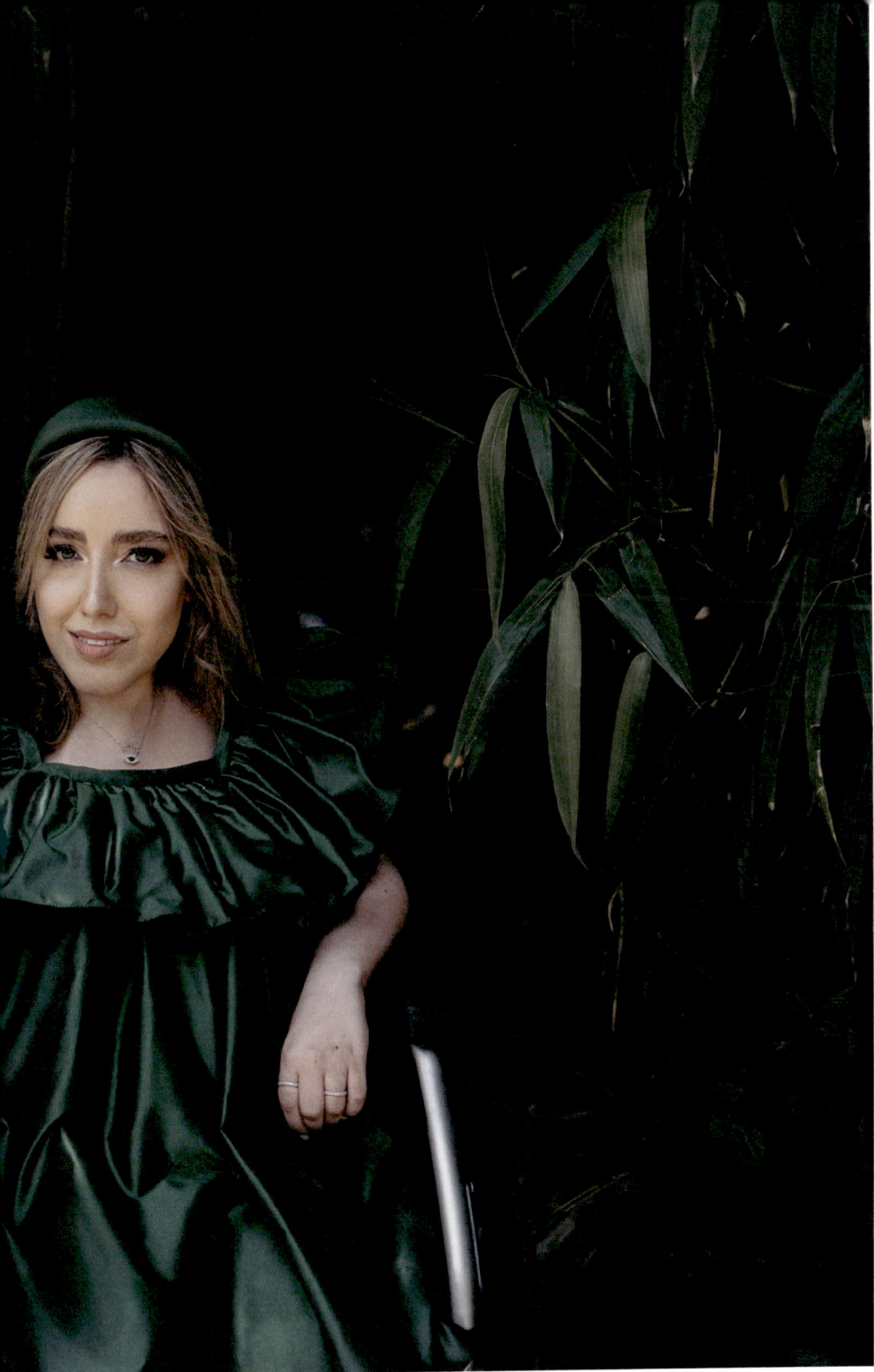

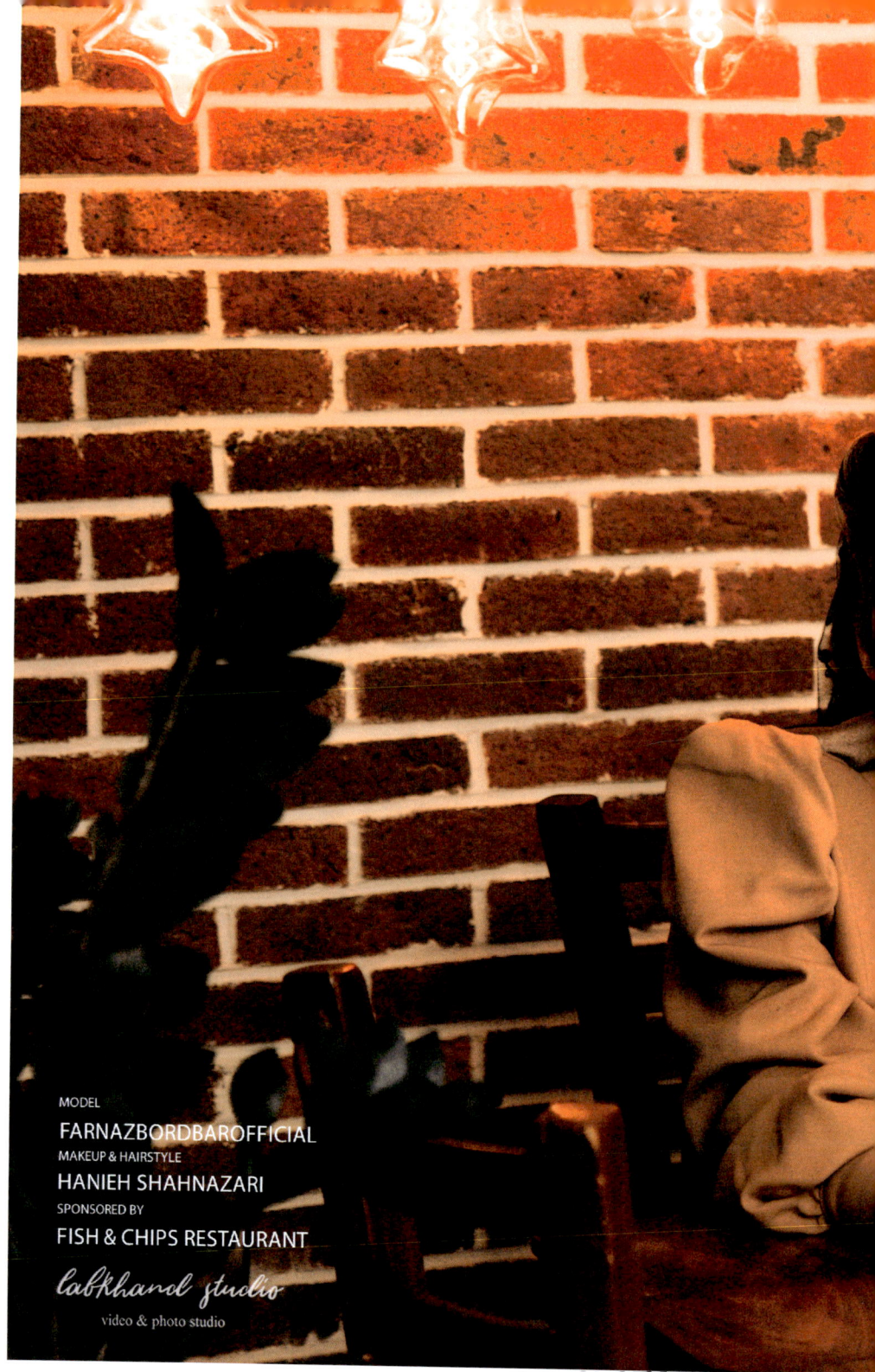

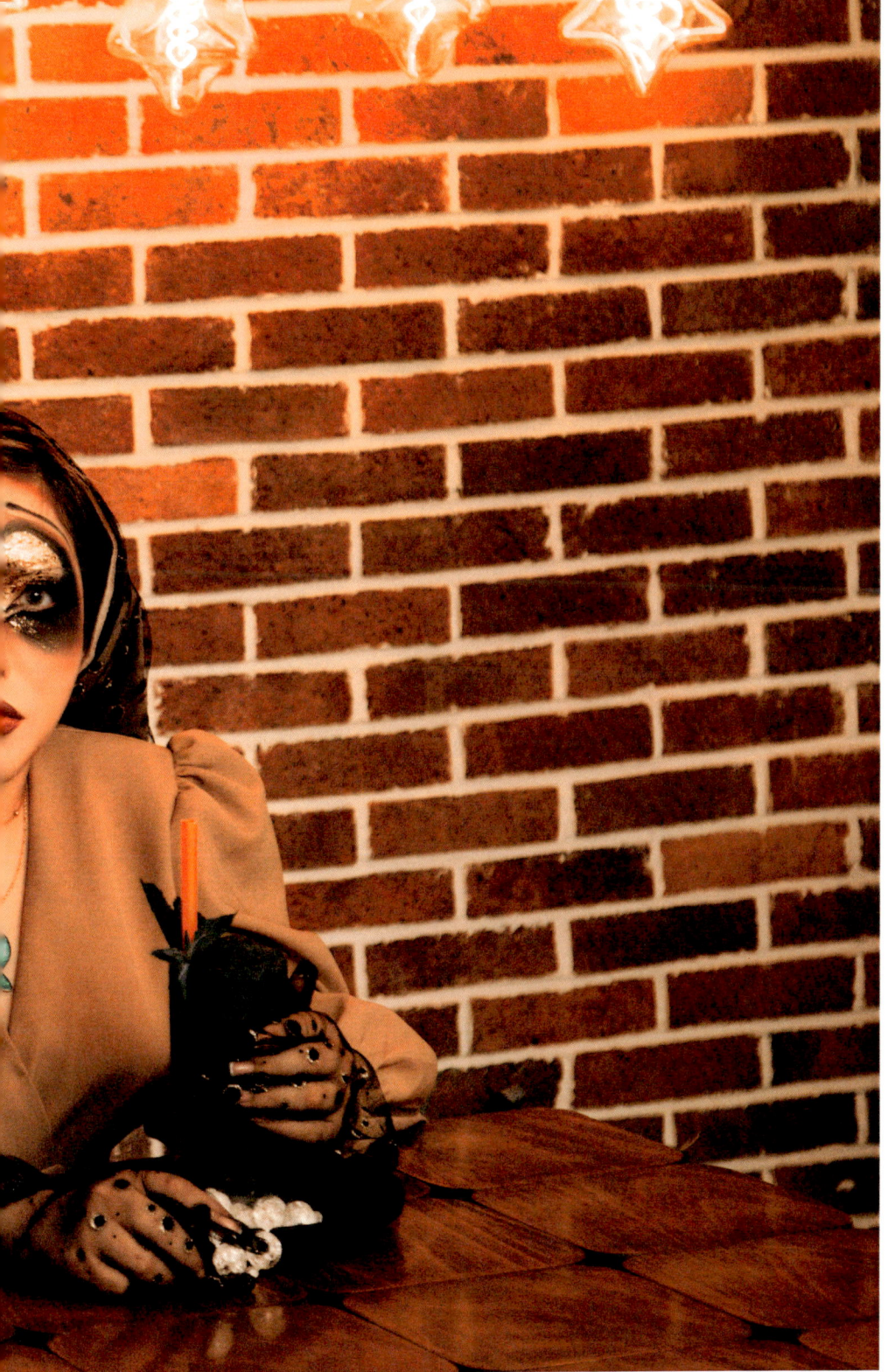

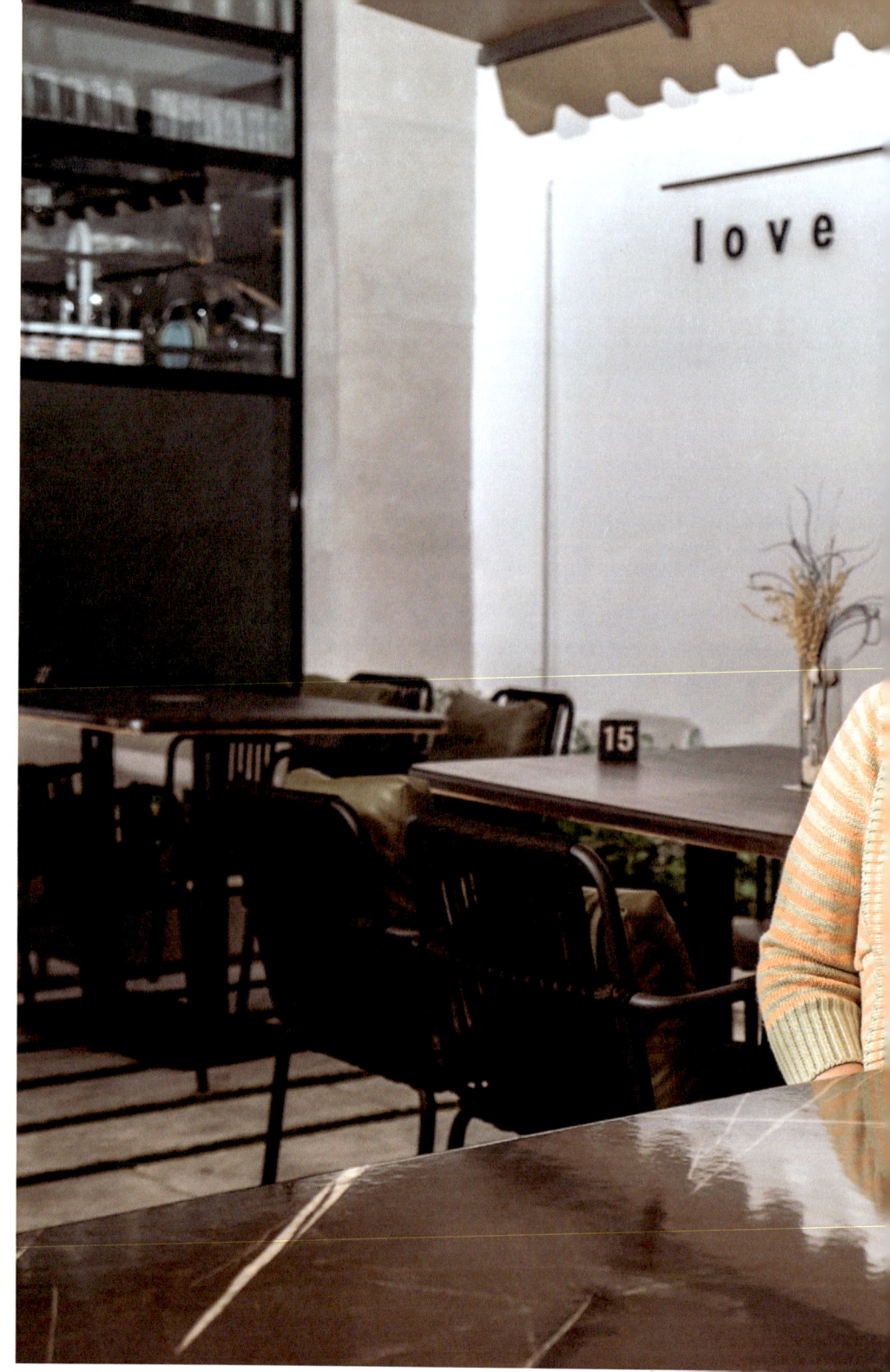

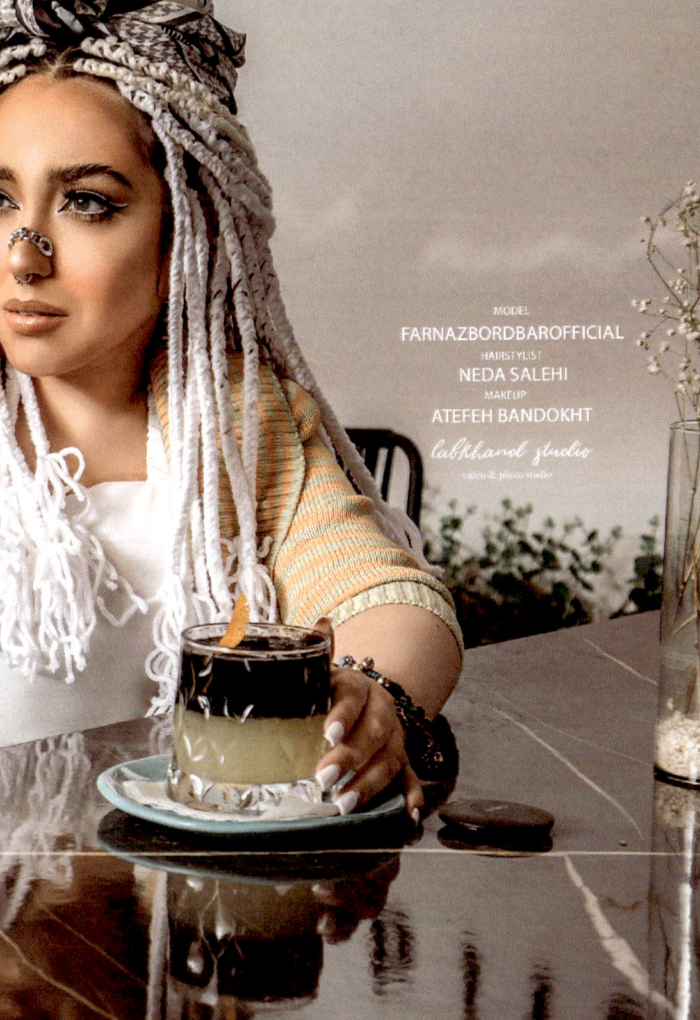

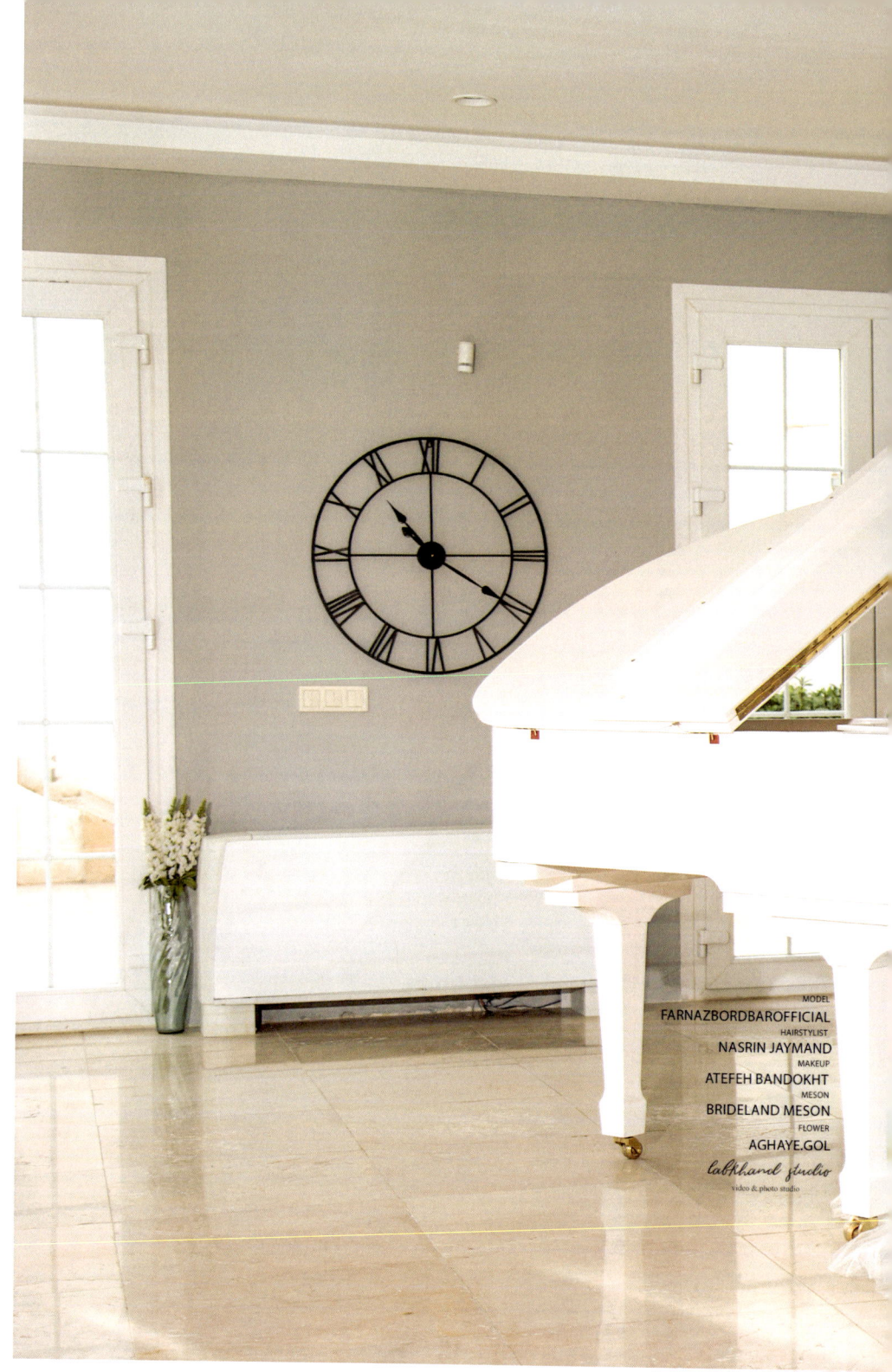

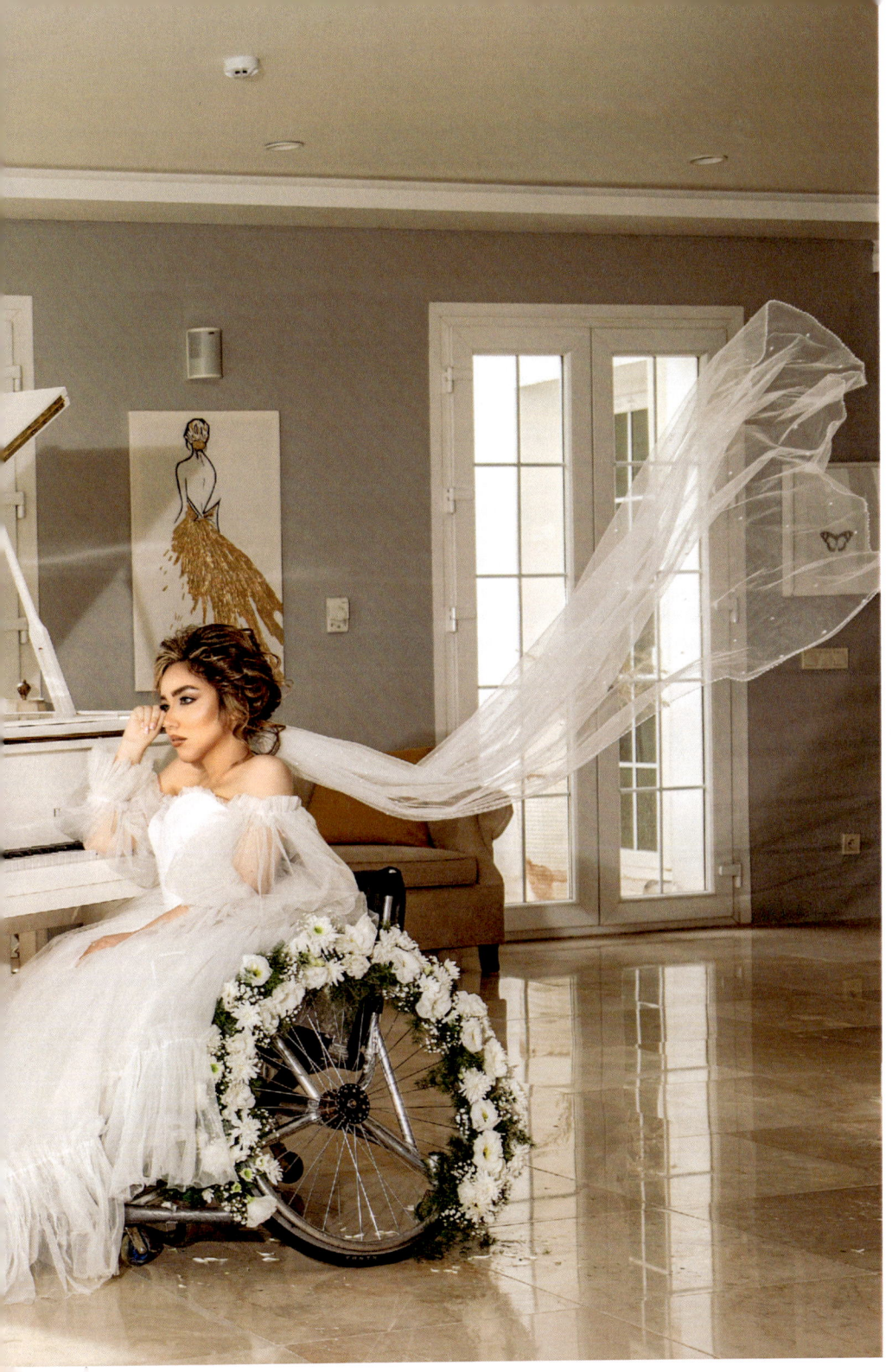

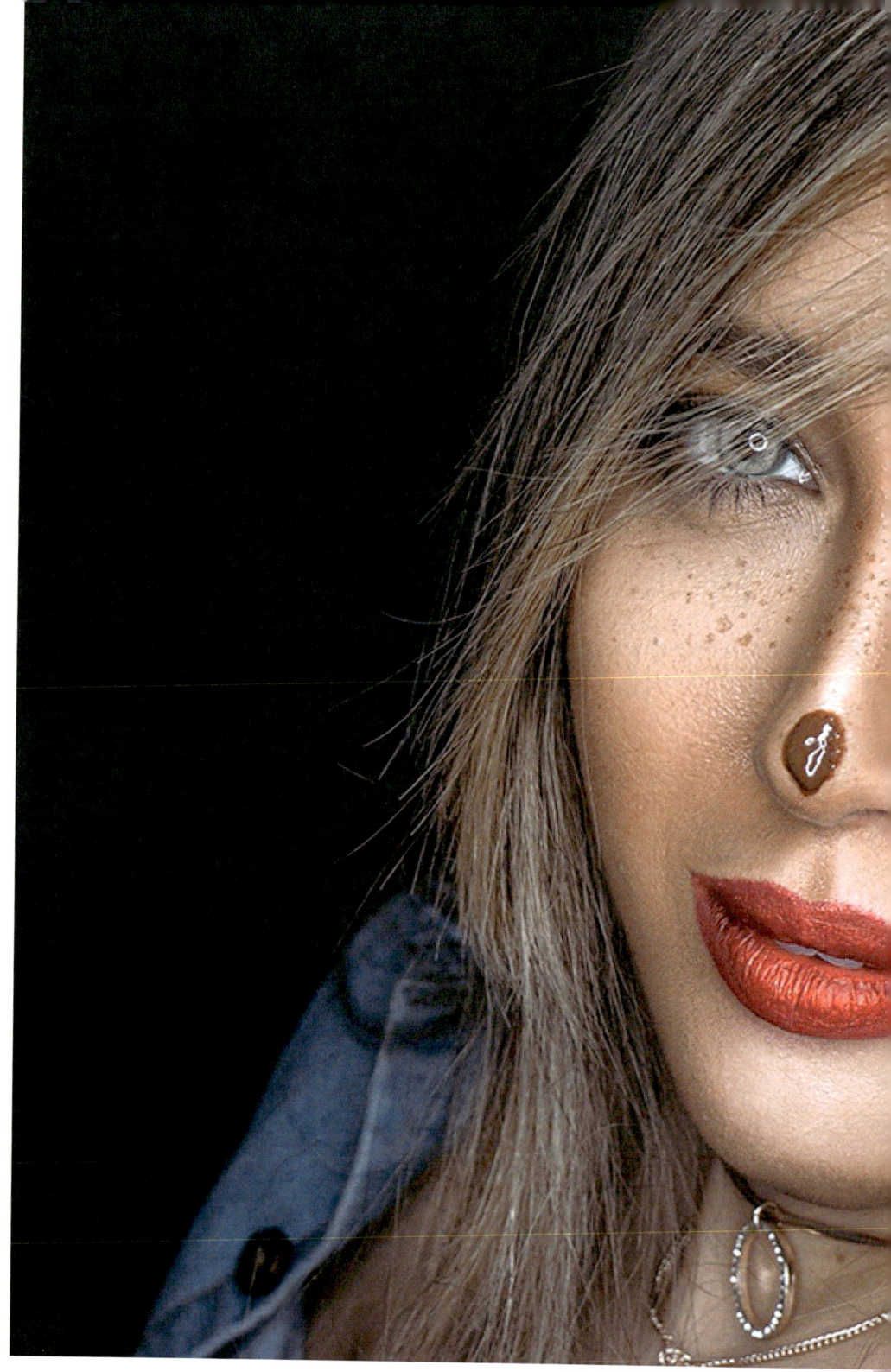

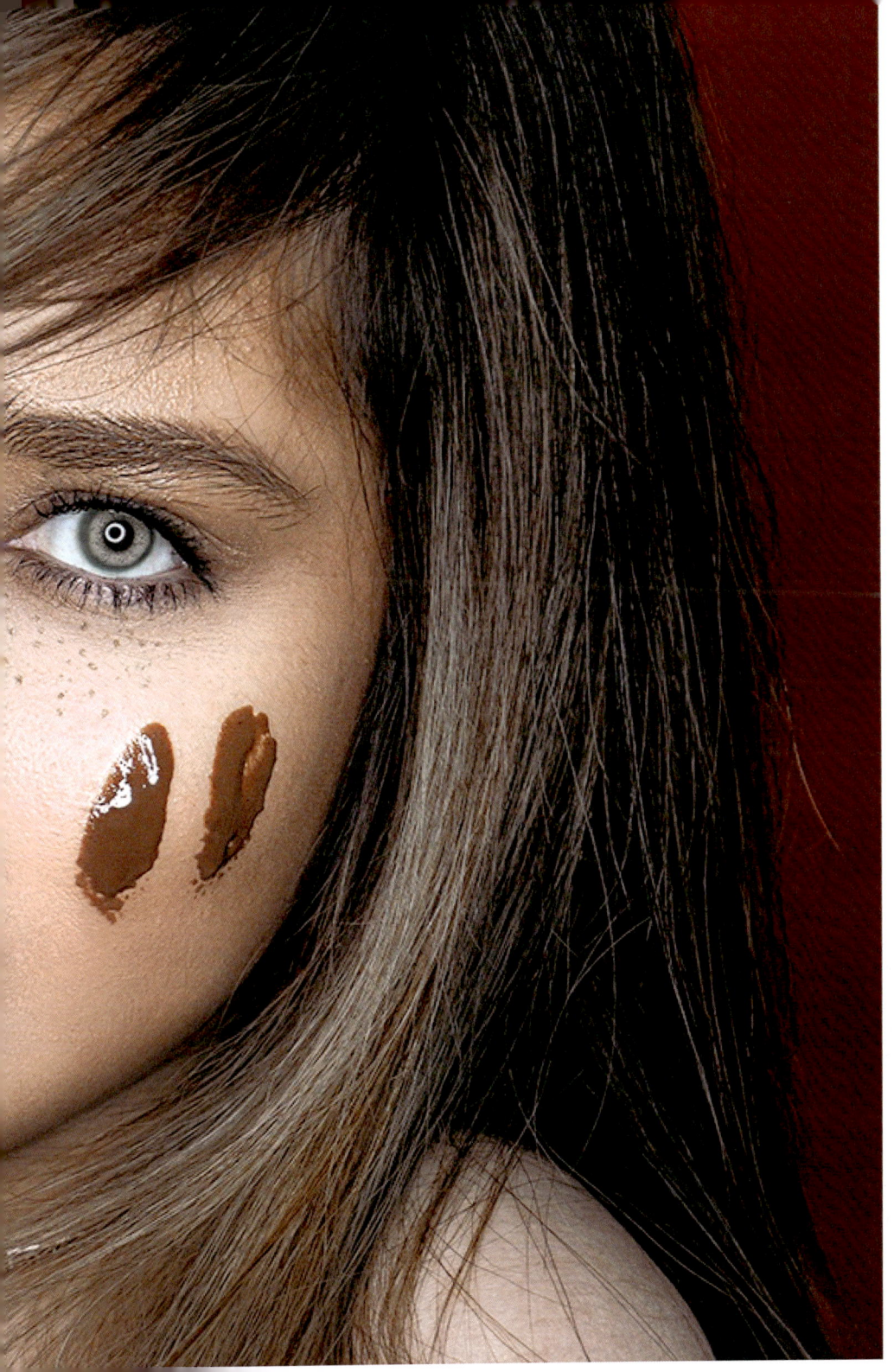

Princess of Chair

www.ingramcontent.com/pod-product-compliance
Lightning Source LLC
Chambersburg PA
CBRC100024110526
44587CB00007BA/159